The Alexander Technique Resource Book

A Reference Guide

John B. Harer
Sharon Munden

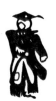

The Scarecrow Press, Inc.
Lanham, Maryland • Toronto • Plymouth, UK
2009

SCARECROW PRESS, INC.

Published in the United States of America
by Scarecrow Press, Inc.
A wholly owned subsidiary of
The Rowman & Littlefield Publishing Group, Inc.
4501 Forbes Boulevard, Suite 200, Lanham, Maryland 20706
www.scarecrowpress.com

Estover Road
Plymouth PL6 7PY
United Kingdom

British Library Cataloguing in Publication Information Available

Library of Congress Cataloging-in-Publication Data
Harer, John B.
  The Alexander technique resource book : a reference guide / John B. Harer, Sharon
Munden.
     p. cm.
  Includes bibliographical references and index.
  ISBN-13: 978-0-8108-5431-4 (pbk. : alk. paper)
  ISBN-10: 0-8108-5431-7 (pbk. : alk. paper)
  ISBN-13: 978-0-8108-6392-7 (ebook)
  ISBN-10: 0-8108-6392-8 (ebook)
   1. Alexander technique–Bibliography. 2. Alexander technique–Directories. I.
Munden, Sharon. II. Title.
  Z6675.A42H37 2009
  [RA781.5]
  016.6137'8–dc22   2008035109

∞™ The paper used in this publication meets the minimum requirements of
American National Standard for Information Sciences—Permanence of Paper
for Printed Library Materials, ANSI/NISO Z39.48-1992.
Manufactured in the United States of America.

Contents

Preface

THE NEED FOR *THE ALEXANDER TECHNIQUE RESOURCE BOOK*

The vocal performance discipline has brought the authors to a rich understanding of the value of the Alexander Technique, not just in the performing arts, but also in many walks of life in and out of the academy. We are often asked, "What is the Alexander Technique?" when we mention our latest project, *The Alexander Technique Resource Book*, most especially in nonperforming arts circles. There is a sense that the technique is not recognized by many people, though other body-work techniques, especially yoga and Pilates, often evince much more understanding as we discuss this technique to enlighten our listeners. Surprisingly, the Alexander Technique has been around for over one hundred years and has helped many famous, and not so famous, individuals with their health and performance, from the author Aldous Huxley to widely popular and famous actors, such as William Hurt and Kevin Kline, both of whom promote the technique in other venues. As a result, the technique should be better known. This book has risen out of the perceived need to close that gap of knowledge about the Alexander Technique, reach a wider audience beyond the performing arts with a wealth of information, and provide a more comprehensive guide to resources on the technique suitable for research and study in a broader array of applications.

There have been some published works that have attempted to provide a similar guide to resources on the Alexander Technique. The limitations of those resources have been another significant reason this book has been developed. The most important of these other resources is *The Reader's Guide to the Alexander Technique: A Selected Annotated Bibliography*, written by Phyllis Sanfilippo and published in 1987. This text has extremely authoritative annotations of the most well-known works about the Alexander Technique, including the seminal works by the technique's pioneers, especially F. M. Alexander (who developed the method), Wilfred Barlow, Frank Pierce Jones, Marjorie Barstow, and Walter Carrington, to mention a few. This work has several limitations that helped determine the need for the current text. Sanfilippo only included ninety-two books and journal articles selected as worthy of being included and annotated, all of which were published before 1987. Many more have been published since 1987, and the more recent resources reflect a broader set of applications of the Alexander Technique in disciplines beyond the performing arts. More importantly, the Internet and electronic resources were not widely available or used prior to the early 1990s, which precluded any coverage by Sanfilippo, and this latest work includes significant resources in electronic form. Sanfilippo's work includes only print resources. Other resources were seen as necessary, especially Internet sites, directories of major schools providing instruction in the technique, and the leading organizations and professional associations of the Alexander Technique.

Additionally, a self-published annotated bibliography, *From Stage-Fright to Seat-Height*, that provides coverage of published works that discuss the Alexander Technique in music applications is available in a few libraries across the country. Prepared by Julia Priest, this brief publication lists less than thirty annotated resources and is limited to subjects relevant to music, including performance anxiety, ergonomics, and musical performance. Having been self-published, it is not widely available. Many books published to explain the Alexander Technique and how it is conducted include a bibliography of sources. These bibliographies are most often not annotated, nor is the coverage significant in number, though they usually include the best works on the technique. This current work has a number of advantages over existing sources. It is much more inclusive than past works. The resources found in this book are current through the first half of 2007 and include materials that have been produced since 1987 when the last resource book was published. The authors have attempted to be more inclusive and provide a much greater number of resources than these earlier sources, though it is not a comprehensive list of all possible publications. The Alexander Technique is largely an international phenomenon that is available in many countries through schools and professional associations, with publications in those languages to inform students and practitioners throughout the world. This work only includes English-language publications that could be acquired through library services in the United States. Lastly, the entries in this book include resources beyond the print world, including electronic resources, audiovisual resources, organizations, and major schools of instruction not included in previous publications.

WHAT THIS BOOK OFFERS YOU

This work is designed as a topical research guide to the Alexander Technique that will provide guidance and information useful for studying the technique and to locate sources for further research in this field. The chapters listing resources are grouped within four broad categories: (1) general works that discuss the efficacy of the technique, how to teach the technique, biographies of well-known Alexander Technique personalities, especially F. M. Alexander, and background information on its development and growth across multiple disciplines; (2) resources for the performing and creative arts; (3) resources for health and medical applications and information; and (4) resources with sports, fitness, and recreation applications. This work begins with an introductory section to describe the history and development of the technique and to provide an understanding of its major principles and methods. Additionally, chapter 6 describes the journals relevant to the Alexander Technique, especially *Direction*, the prime Alexander Technique serial publication, and there are chapters on Internet resources and on directories to Alexander Technique schools and organizations.

Each chapter of annotated, subject-oriented print resources is divided into three sections: (1) books and monographs, (2) journal and magazine articles, and (3) master's and doctoral theses and dissertations. Articles from the popular press that appeal to the general public have been included along with works available from professional journals. Resources were identified through extensive searches of databases providing both general-subject and discipline-specific coverage available from research libraries, especially WorldCat, Academic Search Premier, ProQuest Research, Web of Science, Project Muse, MLA Bibliography, Music Index, and DAI (Dissertations Abstract International), among others. Each resource included in this book was personally examined by the authors for preparation of the annotations. Since other publications listing annotated resources have provided coverage up to 1987, notably Phyllis Sanfilippo's work, only resources published since 1987 have been included, except for the seminal texts by F. M. Alexander and his early protégés, described in the introduction. Each entry in these chapters consists of a complete citation and an annotation of at least two to four hundred words, on the average. The annotations are designed as a review of the work, including description of its structure and design and an explanation of its main content components and ideas, often with some evaluative remarks. The annotations are not designed to describe the resource's content at length.

Chapter 5 on electronic resources also includes annotations for each entry. Chapter 6 on journals relevant to the Alexander Technique is devoted largely to *Direction*, considered the best journal entirely devoted to this technique. This chapter lists every article published in *Direction*. Where the article's content could be identified, a brief annotation has been provided. *Direction* is an Australian publication that is not widely available from American libraries. Several articles could not be examined to provide a plausible annotation. The authors and titles of these articles are listed, however, for each volume. The remaining journal entries in this chapter describe the purpose and coverage of the other journals as they relate to the Alexander Technique. Several of these serial publications are newsletters of various Alexander Technique societies, so no comprehensive attempt to annotate the contents of these volumes has been made. Where articles from these journals could be identified and accessed from a library or electronic resource, they have been annotated and included in the first four chapters, where appropriate. A resource work such as this should include directory information, so chapter 8 has been included listing major schools that teach the Alexander Technique as well as organizations and professional societies devoted to promoting the value of the Alexander Technique.

Acknowledgments

The authors wish to thank the staffs of the Catawba College and East Carolina University libraries for their support and assistance in acquiring the many materials needed for this book, especially two East Carolina University librarians: Lynda Werdal of the Interlibrary Loan department and David Hursh, head of the Music Library. We thank them for their patience, help, and support of this project. We also wish to thank our editor at Scarecrow Press, Martin Dillon, for his encouragement and support of this project. It was invaluable to us when work on the manuscript became difficult.

The authors also wish to acknowledge the invaluable assistance in the development of this book contributed by Martha Fertman of the Philadelphia School for the Alexander Technique. Her advice and counsel has been most invaluable.

Introduction: The History and Foundations of the Alexander Technique

The Alexander Technique is a hands-on educational method to teach individuals to learn how to get rid of unwanted tension in the body, tension that is caused by reactive personal habits and habitual limitations in the way they move and think. Frederick Matthias Alexander, an Australian Shakespearean actor, developed the technique around the turn of the twentieth century (ca. 1890–1904). The Alexander Technique is considered a form of complementary and alternative medicine known as body-work movement therapies within the realm of similar techniques such as Pilates, Feldenkrais, and Rolfing, though it is not as well known as Pilates, particularly, among the general public. The technique is most widely practiced in the performing arts, especially in the theater, film, opera, and dance arenas, and also by other music professions, but has a growing following in other areas, especially the sports and recreational fields of swimming and horseback riding. Some of the world's greatest modern actors, in particular, have greatly benefited from the Alexander Technique, including Kenneth Branagh (*Swing Kids*, *The Gingerbread Man*), John Cleese (*Monty Python's Flying Circus*, *Fawlty Towers*), Kevin Kline (*A Fish Called Wanda*, *Silverado*, *Dave*), and William Hurt (*The Big Chill*, *Kiss of the Spiderwoman*), just to mention a few. The Academy Award winning actor William Hurt has said about the Alexander Technique, "The Alexander Technique has helped me to undo knots, unblock energy, and deal with almost paralyzing stage fright" (Kosminsky and Hurt 1999, liner notes). Kevin Kline, also, has noted,

> The Technique, which seemed at first inexhaustibly mysterious, turned out to be an accessible and most enjoyable discipline to learn and to practice. I have found in the ensuing years, great benefits in my day-to-day living. By balancing and neutralizing tensions, I've learned to relieve as well as avoid the aches and pains caused by the thousands of natural shocks that flesh is heir to. (Leibowitz and Connington 1990, ix)

The most recognized and respected performing arts schools, such as the Julliard School and the Royal College of Music in London, include Alexander Technique training in their curriculum. It was championed in the mid-twentieth century by the well-known British author Sir Aldous Huxley, author of *Brave New World*. Its proponents include the musicians Paul McCartney (the Beatles), Sting (the Police), Julian Bream (classical guitarist), Yehudi Menuhin (violinist and conductor), and James Galway (classical flute). American philosopher John Dewey was a major supporter and proponent of Alexander and his technique.

The benefits of the Alexander Technique have been documented to include improved breathing; relief from back pain; the ability to overcome stage fright; developing greater freedom of movement; improved sports performance in swimming, tennis, and horseback riding; and aid to child birth. However, despite this laudatory record of the technique's impact on many individuals and professions, it is not as well known in the United States, particularly, as other body-work therapies such as Pilates and yoga. This section of the book will introduce the reader to the Alexander Technique's history and development and provide a basic understanding of the technique. Readers should consult the texts listed in the chapters of this book for a more in-depth description of the technique, how it is applied, and its benefits.

THE DISCOVERY AND HISTORICAL DEVELOPMENT
OF THE ALEXANDER TECHNIQUE

Frederick Matthias Alexander, most often cited as "F. M. Alexander," or just "F. M.," was an Australian who made his initial reputation as a Shakespearean reciter and actor. A "Shakespearean reciter" provided a form of dramatic entertainment, considered a form of oratory emphasizing the use of elocution, where one person performed soliloquies, well-known speeches, or parts of a Shakespearean play. During the late 1800s, English-speaking countries highly valued oratorical skills due to the rise of parliaments whose members relied upon political oratory for electoral and legislative successes. In our American tradition, for example, the great orators of the period included Henry Clay, Daniel Webster, and, of course, Abraham Lincoln. Oratorical skills became a common form of entertainment as well, rivaling dramatic productions. For instance, Emerson College, considered one of the premier colleges for theater arts today, was founded in 1880 by Charles Emerson, a Unitarian minister, as the Boston Conservatory of Elocution, Oratory, and Dramatic Art because of Emerson's belief in the value of oratorical skill. Shakespearean oratory, or recitation, was one type of this popular, oratorical entertainment. Additionally, the Chautauqua and Lyceum movements of the late 1800s and early 1900s provided Shakespearean recitation as part of their entertainment venue. To the Chautauqua movement, Shakespeare's works were seen as popular crowd pleasers but the plays, in their entirety, too risqué for their mostly rural and conservative audience, so more often, individual speeches or edited portions of Shakespeare's work were performed or recited.

The roots of Alexander's family, however, were British farmers. According to his biographer, J. A. Evans, a grandnephew, he was the grandson of Matthias Alexander, a hurdle maker, who was forced to leave England for his part in the Captain Swing Riots of 1830. These riots were part of a larger agrarian revolution against the mechanization of farming, especially against the introduction of the thresher, which caused much rural poverty through the loss of jobs when farmers switched harvest production to the thresher (Evans 2001). Matthias and his brother John, a carpenter, were sentenced to "transportation" for seven years, a term for banishment to another area of the realm, with Matthias ending up in Stanley, Tasmania. F. M. Alexander was born in 1869 on a farm in Tasmania. Due to ill health, mainly respiratory problems, he was sent to private school for his early education. In his teens, his formal education ended after his family moved to a mining town due to financial difficulties. F.M. then worked at educating himself while working many odd jobs, training in drama and in music with local teachers. In these experiences, he became fascinated with reciting through his love of poetry. In his book *The Use of the Self*, Alexander said, "From my early youth I took a delight in poetry and it was one of my chief pleasures to study the plays of Shakespeare, reading them aloud and endeavoring to interpret the characters. This led to my becoming interested in elocution and the art of reciting" (Alexander 1932, 6). He eventually moved to Melbourne where he continued his own path of education for the theater arts, developing a reputation by his midtwenties for producing Shakespearean plays and recitals and as a Shakespearean reciter and actor in his own right.

By the early 1890s, Alexander began having great difficulty on stage with severe hoarseness. During his recitals, friends would tell him that he would begin gasping and sucking in air, worsening over time to the point where he would lose his voice entirely during a recital. The medical advice at the time was primarily a prescription for rest between performances, yet after resting for more than two weeks prior to a very important engagement, his hoarseness returned so severely halfway through the performance that he lost his voice. This event caused Alexander to question and then reject conventional medical advice for his problem. It was this questioning that began his journey into self-discovery of the misuse of his body.

> When I set out on this investigation, I had two facts to go on. I had learned that reciting brought about conditions of hoarseness, and that this hoarseness tended to disappear, as long as I confined the use of my voice to ordinary speaking, and at the same time had medical treatment for my throat and vocal organs. I considered the bearing of these two facts upon my difficulty, and I saw that if ordinary speaking did not cause hoarseness while reciting did, there must be something different between what I did in reciting and what I did in ordinary speaking. (Alexander 1932, 9)

He devised a plan for examining himself while reciting, observing how he spoke and how he held his head before a mirror. Over time, he found what he described as his "manner of doing," three distinct issues in the way he spoke and recited: (1) a stiffening of the neck that retracted his head, which he described as "pulling the head back"; (2) depression of his larynx; and (3) a sucking in of his breath with a kind of gasp (Gelb 1981). Throughout Alexander's self-discovery process, he gradually changed his view of the relationship between the mind and the body. He had, much like many people, viewed them as separate, working independently. But, later, as he notes in *The Use of the Self*, he came to the conclusion that "it is *impossible* (Alexander's emphasis) to separate 'mental' and 'physical' processes in any form of human activity" (Alexander 1932, 3). After these initial discoveries, Alexander came to realize the need to create a method for controlling his voice consistently, so he increased the number of mirrors for further observation. Frank Pierce Jones noted,

> He realized that his response to the stimulus to speak was indeed a total pattern, for it involved an increase in muscle tension everywhere. To deal with the problem, he devised a set of "directions" (messages from the brain to the various mechanisms) for relaxing the muscles in his neck instead of tensing them, allowing his head to go "forward and up" instead of pulling it backward and down, lengthening his spine instead of arching it, and widening his back instead of narrowing it. (Jones 1976, 17)

Alexander's self-discovery process evolved over several years in the 1890s. During this time frame, he continued to work as a reciter and actor, while also building a practice of teaching what he had learned as a technique. In addition to aiding people in the performing arts, his reputation encouraged some Australian doctors to send other patients his way with much success. His reputation for the healing qualities of his technique grew, despite suspicions in the medical profession as a whole. By 1904, a prominent surgeon, J. W. Steward McKay, who had become an enthusiastic patron, encouraged him to move to London to build a greater and more international impact. As Michael Gelb notes, "In London, Alexander's practice developed rapidly, and he soon became known as 'the protector of the London theatre,'" giving lessons and gaining high praise from London's professional acting class, among others (Gelb 1981, 15). By 1910, there was evidence of a number of imitators, many of whom practiced improper forms of the technique. Alexander published his first book, *Man's Supreme Inheritance*, in part to protect the sanctity of his work from plagiarism and to set an accurate record of the technique's methods. In 1914, Alexander's practice dwindled due to a shortage of patients from the impact of World War I's demand on manpower in England, so he moved to the United States, where his practice also flourished. For ten years, he traveled back and forth between the UK and the United States, building a greater reputation and number of admirers and supporters. Among his many U.S. supporters was John Dewey, the philosopher and educator, who became a pupil of Alexander's and who wrote introductions to three of Alexander's books, including for *The Use of the Self*. Alexander also taught a number of prominent British personalities who became enthusiastic supporters, including the playwright George Bernard Shaw and, especially, the author Aldous Huxley. Huxley, by then a well-known novelist, met Alexander in the mid-1930s. At that time, however, he was virtually bedridden from chronic fatigue, insomnia, and a weak stomach, causing him to fall into a deep depression. Alexander administered his technique, which vastly improved Huxley's health for the remainder of his life. Alexander's work made such a remarkable change in Huxley that he was able to complete the novel *Eyeless in Gaza*, which had been languishing due to his ill health, creating the character "Miller" in the story, a medical anthropologist, modeled after Alexander (Jones 1976).

Though Alexander firmly believed as Dewey did that education was the key to social evolution and success, he did not establish a formal training course until 1930. Schools for children based on the technique did exist in the 1920s, especially from the efforts of Irene Tasker, a protégé of Maria Montessori as well as Alexander. Alexander was inspired to develop his three-year curriculum for teachers of the technique after the experiences of his brother, Albert Redden Alexander, also known as "A.R." A.R., an avid horseman, had a serious riding accident that had crushed his spine. Doctors at the time told him he would never walk again, but A.R. rigorously practiced his brother's technique into a full recovery. This was the impetus for the formal training course now in use today. A.R. became one of the most prominent Alexander Technique teachers in the United States in the 1930s and 1940s.

F. M. Alexander continued to teach and write about his technique, even after a severe stroke in 1948 that paralyzed his left side, until he passed away in 1955. He used his technique to overcome the debilitating effects of his stroke. During the 1930s and 1940s, he published two books: *The Use of the Self* (1932) and *The Universal Constant in Living* (1941). However, a significant controversy in 1948 threatened all of his life's work. His theories and ideas were attacked vociferously by Dr. Ernst Jokl, director of the South African Physical Education Committee, after Alexander's supporters attempted to integrate his technique into a physical education curriculum for South African schools. Alexander sued for libel and, with the support of the Nobel Prize winning neurophysiologist Sir Charles Sherrington and the noted anthropologist Raymond Dart, successfully defended his technique in the trial.

Alexander's work has not stopped with his passing. As Gelb notes, "Alexander's achievement was immense. He developed, on his own, an entirely new scientific method of examining and solving a particular problem and in so doing established a revolutionary way of looking at human functioning" (Gelb 1981, 19–20). Many knowledgeable people, such as Gelb, have noted that Alexander and his work are not as well known as other techniques in the body-work movement, especially Pilates, which has been seen as parallel in a number of ways. Many scholars of the technique, among them Gelb, have speculated that this was due to Alexander's personality and his insistence on extremely high standards, reducing the factors that would promote the technique more widely. Despite this, the Alexander Technique has gained widespread acceptance and notoriety, in particular since the 1970s, especially as more teachers have been trained and as more people have been helped by the Alexander Technique.

THE PUBLISHED WORKS OF FREDERICK MATTHIAS ALEXANDER

Anyone wishing to learn more about the Alexander Technique would do well to examine the four major works of F. M. Alexander. These books constitute Alexander's ideas and thinking about the technique, how it was developed, its benefits to mankind, and how it is applied. The four works were written between 1910 and 1941, beginning with *Man's Supreme Inheritance*, published at a time when there were many counterfeit techniques based on his work being touted as truly Alexander Technique methods. His next two books reflect how the technique evolved over time, introducing and explaining other principles of the technique. His final work is a collection of articles and essays on various aspects and topics of the technique.

Man's Supreme Inheritance (New York: Dutton, 1910)

The major theme of this book is to describe the "great phase in Man's advancement in which he passes from subconscious to conscious control of his own mind and body." The title represents Alexander's view that reason and intelligence drive man's choices. He makes a clear case for the concept that humans function as a whole body, mental and physical functions intertwined and interrelated. This is Alexander's philosophy of human nature, and his technique is explained thoroughly as he had devised it up to that point. Phyllis Sanfilippo (1987) states that it is "important for gaining insight into Alexandrian thinking" but criticizes its limitations as "suffer[ing] from verbal convolutions and complexities in an effort to describe kinesthesia" (Sanfilippo 1987, 12).

Constructive Conscious Control of the Individual (London: Methuen, 1923)

Alexander's second book, this text introduces the concepts of "end-gaining" and "sensory application." It also was one of the earliest lists of procedures used in a typical lesson, in considerable detail. In this work, Alexander attempted to answer some questions that arose after writing *Man's Supreme Inheritance*, with an emphasis on the unity between body and mind. Alexander also devotes some discussion to the difficulty of describing the kinesthetic self and action in words, noting, "We cannot write a kinesthesia any more than we can write the sense of sound" (Alexander 1923, 77).

The Use of the Self (New York: Dutton, 1932)

This is Alexander's account of how he discovered his technique, and it also introduces the terms "use" and "primary control." Alexander uses two "case histories" to illustrate the principles he describes in the book, including (1) the golfer who cannot keep his eye on the ball and (2) the stutterer. Alexander also discusses issues of medical diagnosis and treatment. John Dewey wrote an introduction to this book.

The Universal Constant in Living (New York: Dutton, 1947)

This is Alexander's last book and contains numerous articles, case histories, letters, and quotes from other books, papers, and journalistic reports on various topics Alexander wished to explain in some detail. It includes an unpublished essay by Aldous Huxley and an introduction by George E. Coghill, a biologist. Sanfilippo notes that "it stresses Alexander's theme of unity within the individual which is emphasized throughout the work" (Sanfilippo 1987, 12).

There have been numerous works published during Alexander's lifetime that also play a role in furthering the Alexander Technique and in aiding its dissemination worldwide, most notably from some of Alexander's contemporaries and followers during the mid-twentieth century, including Frank Pierce Jones, Wilfred Barlow, Walter Carrington, and Patrick Macdonald. This book has not attempted to include these other works but has focused on resources published or created since 1987. The resources published before 1987 have been thoroughly documented by Phyllis Sanfilippo in her book *The Reader's Guide to the Alexander Technique: A Selected Annotated Bibliography*. Her book includes substantial annotations and explanations of the contents of these works. The reader should consult Sanfilippo's book in addition to this current text for a more complete guide to the literature on the Alexander Technique.

IMPORTANT CONTEMPORARIES AND PROTÉGÉS

The Alexander Technique could not have been advanced in its early years without support from other individuals. Alexander gained a number of supporters who believed in his work, some of whom became teachers of the technique, and all of whom contributed in some way to its dissemination and longevity as a beneficial technique. A study of these individuals and their work is also important for understanding the technique's history, development, and use. The most prominent individuals are listed, but by no means is this to be considered an exhaustive list.

Albert Redden Alexander (1874–1947)

Also known as "A.R.," he was one of F.M.'s nine brothers and sisters, five years his junior. A.R. became a prominent and well-known Alexander Technique teacher. It was his work with John Dewey that gained Dewey's support for the technique. A.R. joined F.M. early on in the practice of the technique, following F.M. to London in 1907. Numerous chroniclers of the Alexander Technique have noted how Alexander was inspired by A.R.'s use of the technique to overcome a crushed spine from a terrible horseback riding accident. A.R. moved permanently to the United States, first to Boston in the 1930s after the death of his wife, then later to Media, Pennsylvania. He remained a noted Alexander Technique teacher there until his death in 1947 while visiting his brother in England.

Wilfred (1915–1993) and Marjory Barlow (1915–2006)

Wilfred and Marjory Barlow were early and well-known teachers of the Alexander Technique who helped maintain a strict legacy of Alexander's teaching methods and beliefs well into the 1990s. Marjory was F. M. Alexander's niece, daughter of his sister Amy. She entered F.M.'s first Alexander Technique teacher training course in 1932, becoming fully certified as a teacher in 1936. Wilfred, a rheumatologist, met Marjory in 1940 when he became interested in the medical benefits of the technique. Wilfred wrote the book *The Alexander Principle*, one of the most well-known works on the technique. Marjory later became the chairperson of the Society of Teachers of the Alexander Technique (STAT), the UK's professional association for the Alexander Technique. In her later years, she was noted for advocating for the purity of Alexander's legacy. She recorded, with Trevor Allan Davies, audio recordings of Alexander's four books.

Marjorie Barstow (1899–1995)

Marjorie Barstow was the first certified teacher of the Alexander Technique, entering F.M.'s school in 1933 and becoming certified in 1934. Marjorie began her career as a teacher and as A. R. Alexander's assistant in Boston. During these years, she met and befriended Frank Pierce Jones, and their friendship lasted until Jones's death in 1975. Barstow was originally from Lincoln, Nebraska, and moved back there in the early 1950s. She was offered a teaching post at the University of Nebraska and conducted courses and training in the Midwest for the remainder of her life. She taught and influenced some of the most respected and well-known teachers today, including Bruce Fertman and Martha Hansen Fertman, Michael and Lena Frederick, and William and Barbara Conable. Her work can be found in the book *Marjorie Barstow: Her Teaching and Training*, by Barbara Conable (Columbus, Ohio: Andover Road Press, 1989).

Walter H. M. Carrington (1915–2005)

Carrington was one of the earliest and most well-known teachers of the Alexander Technique. Though he originally planned to become a member of the

Society of Jesus, he became so impressed by how the technique had aided his mother that he began taking lessons as well, eventually entering Alexander's teacher training course in 1936. In 1940, he married Dilys Jones, who joined him as a teacher for the remainder of their lives. After a tour of duty as an RAF pilot during World War II, he returned to practice as an Alexander Technique teacher in numerous locations throughout Great Britain. After Alexander's death in 1955, he and three other teachers carried on Alexander's teacher training course, developing it into the Constructive Teaching Centre. He is also widely known for two books of lectures on the technique, *Thinking Aloud* (1994) and *The Act of Living* (1999), as well as the book *Explaining the Alexander Technique: The Writings of F. M. Alexander* (1992).

Aldous Huxley (1894–1963)

Huxley is one of the most famous authors in English literature, especially noted for his novel *Brave New World*. However, his connection to F. M. Alexander and his technique is also very significant. The Wikipedia© (online encyclopedia) article on Huxley lists F. M. Alexander as one of three influences on Huxley's life. The two met in 1935 when Huxley sought him for his worsening condition of chronic fatigue, insomnia, and a weak stomach, which had led to a deep depression. Alexander's ministrations vastly improved Huxley's health to the point where even his reluctance for public speaking improved. During this time, Huxley had been struggling to complete his novel *Eyeless in Gaza*. As his health improved, he found an ending to the novel that had previously escaped him by creating the character "Miller," a medical anthropologist, modeled after Alexander. Huxley then went on to write the philosophical work *Ends and Means*, which was directly influenced by Alexander's teachings and his technique. Huxley became a leading supporter and advocate of the technique. His last novel, *Island* (1960), considered a utopian novel, was also heavily influenced by Alexander's work.

Frank Pierce Jones (1905–1975)

Frank Pierce Jones was a prominent advocate of the Alexander Technique, especially in the United States. He is the author of *Body Awareness in Action: A Study of the Alexander Technique* that includes descriptions of his experimental studies at Tufts University, and elsewhere, that were designed to show a scientific basis for the technique. Jones held a PhD in the Classics from the University of Wisconsin at Madison and became a professor of Greek and Latin at Brown University in the early 1930s. He had suffered from severe allergies all of his life and, during this period, contracted tuberculosis. While resigned to the debilitating effects of tuberculosis for a few years, he came to read Aldous Huxley's *Ends and Means*, Huxley's 1938 work touting the Alexander Technique. After lessons with

A. R. Alexander vastly improved his health, Jones became a committed advocate and eventually a teacher of the technique, taking lessons with F.M. during the 1940s war years. Jones later developed experimental techniques to test various principles of the Alexander Technique in a laboratory setting, working with the Tufts Institute of Applied Experimental Psychology for the rest of his career.

Patrick Macdonald (1910–1992)

Macdonald was also an early member of F. M. Alexander's first teacher training course, beginning his work with the curriculum in 1933. He was a lifelong teacher and advocate of the technique until his death in 1992. He is noted particularly for his book *The Alexander Technique as I See It* (Brighton, UK: Rahula Books, 1989). This work is a collection of articles and essays by Macdonald from his experiences with the technique.

WHY THE ALEXANDER TECHNIQUE IS BENEFICIAL

Historically, there have been numerous anecdotal accounts of how the Alexander Technique has vastly improved one's health and life, from many famous individuals as well as ordinary students of Alexander teachers worldwide. We know that Aldous Huxley, author of *Brave New World*, suffered greatly from chronic fatigue, insomnia, and a deep mental depression until he found that the technique was able to vastly improve his health. Frank Pierce Jones, who did extensive research on the technique at Tufts University, suffered greatly from severe allergies as well as tuberculosis until the Alexander Technique allowed him to rehabilitate himself. As mentioned earlier, the Academy Award winning actor, William Hurt, found that the Alexander Technique helped him overcome stage fright, a malady that could kill an actor's career. Different anecdotes show that the technique has benefits in numerous areas. Less well-known people have also testified to how the Alexander Technique saved them from debilitating pain or other health problems. Hugh Massey, a noted anthropologist, contracted tuberculosis while completing research in Africa and was cured through the use of the technique. Judith Leibowitz, one of the more well-known experts on the Alexander Technique, was introduced to it as an acting student while at the Julliard School. She had been stricken with polio in her teen years, paralyzed from the waist down, until conventional physical therapy restored use of her limbs, though leaving her with a limp. After intensive work with the Alexander Technique in just the initial training period, she noted, "The improvement that took place in my body during that month was dramatic. My limp improved greatly. My body began to straighten out its distortions, and I moved more easily" (Leibowitz and Connington 1990, 5). Steven Shaw, a noted swimming instructor and inventor of the Shaw Method of Swimming, discovered from his use of the

Alexander Technique that it greatly improved his ability in competitive swimming. Also, Paul Collins, a noted marathon runner, found that the Alexander Technique restored his ability to run after suffering debilitating injuries. Emma Kirkby, a world-renowned classical singer, found the technique improved her ability to sing and perform on stage. Alec McCowen, a British actor, has said that it vastly improved his pain from arthritis and back trouble. Countless lesser-known individuals have testified to the great benefit of the Alexander Technique in their lives as well. In fact, many texts on the Alexander Technique as well as many websites that feature it include testimonials from the famous as well as the average Alexander Technique student.

While the anecdotal record may not be considered scientific evidence, these accounts point to what many people see as the type of benefits of the Alexander Technique. They show that it can improve or cure breathing problems and diseases associated with breathing difficulties, such as allergies or tuberculosis. The technique has been seen as capable of improving or eliminating pain from back trouble, arthritis, and sports injuries. The Alexander Technique has been known to aid people with other body and movement problems, such as Leibowitz's work to improve her limp brought on by polio, or Albert Redden Alexander's recovery from a crushed spine due to a horseback riding injury. Some of the most well-known actors, musicians, and dancers of our time, from all forms of these arts, have touted the technique's benefits in performance, including facilitating acting, ease of stage movement, and improved singing, as well as the ability to overcome stage fright. Numerous sports figures and instructors have found that the Alexander Technique increases sports performance, especially in swimming, tennis, golf, and horseback riding. There is a growing body of literature showing the benefits of the technique for aiding childbirth as well.

As F. M. Alexander discovered, many of the conditions that this technique can improve are borne from the fact that unwanted tension, especially systemic long-term tension, from the way we walk, sit, stand, breathe, and do just about any activity causes numerous physical difficulties, especially back and neck pain. Alexander and others discovered that we produce reflexive responses from habits learned through our childhood, extending through adulthood through unconscious repetition of those habitual ways of doing things. In so doing, this tension causes stress on joints, bones, muscles, and the body in general that under extreme misuse can contribute to or even cause pain and other difficulties. Several works have documented that babies and toddlers sit, stand, and move naturally and that, through watching and imitating adults and through the learning process as they mature, they develop inefficient use of the body, losing that innate, natural movement ability over time. For example, toddlers lift objects to their faces whereas habitual use more often finds us bending over them to see. Toddlers squat down to pick up an object instead of bending over to pick the object up. Once in school, this acculturation to inefficient habitual use continues and adds stress to the gathering body tensions. The stress comes from sitting long hours and from a culture of focusing on working hard to learn to be a good student, which adds more stress. As Leibowitz says,

> The child brings the same attitudes and stresses to every new discipline (e.g., dance, sports, music). Physical and emotional stress, cultural demands, imitation, and patterns of thought are among the elements that can lead to a pattern of habitual movement that is inefficient, tension producing, and often painful and which can distort the musculoskeletal system. (Leibowitz and Connington 1990, 38)

There are widespread benefits for physical and emotional health that have been identified in numerous venues, especially by teachers and scholars of the Alexander Technique, and from Alexander students' individual accounts. People become more aware of the use of their body and learn to reduce or eliminate the stress on neck, back, joints, and muscles. It improves balance, ease of movement, and stamina, so often needed in sports and in performance arts. Some proponents of the Alexander Technique believe that it can improve thinking ability, reduce emotional stress, and improve a sense of self. Alexander himself made significant arguments that the mind and body are linked and cannot operate one without the other. Several authors of works on the Alexander Technique, such as Alex Maunder, argue that it shows people that the core of our being is the flow carrying the person physically, mentally, and emotionally. More specific benefits have been noted in health fields and especially accepted in medical circles in the United Kingdom where the Alexander Technique enjoys a greater reputation. The United Kingdom National Health Service recognizes the Alexander Technique as a complementary and alternative medicine, which means that the technique is effective used in conjunction with other, more traditional medical treatments. It acknowledges the benefits under these conditions for back problems, improving ergonomics, reducing or eliminating stuttering and other forms of speech rehabilitation, loss of voice, aiding sufferers of Parkinson's disease, improving posture or balance problems, or adding to and complementing the benefits of physical therapy. The benefits in the performing arts are myriad and diverse. Actors report freer stage movement ability and the ability to overcome stage fright, as well as enhancing the ability to project the voice. Voice and breathing benefits aid opera performers as well. Musicians report the ability to breathe better and more efficiently, which improves musical performance, and to sit or stand more efficiently. Dancers show marked improvement in stretching the torso and improving stress on legs, feet, and joints. In sports and recreational fields, the lengthening or stretching of the torso, aided by lessons in the Alexander Technique, greatly improves swimming and running techniques and ability.

To study the Alexander Technique, however, is not a simple process. It is not accessible as a self-taught method. Some other body-work methods, such as Pilates, can be learned on one's own through reading books and watching videos of the method. This may be one of the reasons the Alexander Technique is not in widespread use in the United States. It requires work with a trained, certified teacher. The Alexander Technique is a hands-on teaching process that requires the instructor to place his or her hands on the student's body, especially the back, neck, and shoulder, while giving verbal instruction. In some Asian cultures, a cultural prohibition on touching has made it difficult to introduce the technique in those countries. Furthermore, while more urban areas have options for locating a teacher, some rural areas are limited in what teachers are available to provide lessons. These lessons with an instructor are time consuming and require a considerable amount of time to complete a full therapy, most often twenty to forty lessons. The technique emphasizes what Alexander called "undoing." Frank Pierce Jones stated, "For the Alexander Technique doesn't teach you something new to do. It teaches you how to bring more practical intelligence into what you are already doing; how to eliminate stereo-typed responses; how to deal with habit and change" (Jones 1997, 2). In other words, it is not a process of learning a new way of behaving, acting, or moving but rather a process to unlearn old habits. This has, in some individuals, triggered unpleasant or unresolved emotional issues. Furthermore, some of the ingrained habits can linger and be impossible or near impossible to undo in some individuals. For some medical conditions, such as arthritis and Parkinson's disease, the technique cannot cure or remove the basic conditions of the disease but merely aid in the comfort of the individual, which can greatly reduce the self-limiting effects of these conditions.

THE ALEXANDER TECHNIQUE

As all publications about the Alexander Technique emphasize, it is a hands-on system that must be administered by a trained Alexander instructor. It cannot be self-taught or learned on one's own from reading a book or viewing a video. Many individuals have described how difficult it is to explain in simple terms, including F. M. Alexander himself, who wrote, "We cannot write a kinesthesia any more than we can write the sense of sound" (Alexander 1923, 77). As mentioned earlier, the actor Kevin Kline found it "inexhaustibly mysterious" when first taking lessons on the technique. Any attempt to fully illustrate the Alexander Technique poses serious difficulties. The reader should realize that any description of the technique should be undertaken as a means to begin a comprehension of it, then accompany that with a lesson or more to fully grasp the technique and how it works. A thorough explication of what might be understood from reading about the technique in its fullest sense is beyond the scope of this text. However, an understanding of the basic principles of the Alexander Technique will provide anyone a point from which to begin their exploration of it and whether or not it would be beneficial.

To begin to discern the basic principles, it is best to examine how unwanted tensions that cause pain and other physical difficulties occur. Such an understanding will aid the reader in conceiving how and why the basic principles work. This is where Alexander began his explorations into his own pain, and how the technique was developed. Habits can be beneficial, some action that always leads to maximizing the functions of the self, such as a regimen for sleep or rest. Habits also can be damaging, actions that hurt the individual through constant repetition, such as the way one would type, drive a car, or walk favoring one foot over the other. Habits can be consciously acted upon or totally unconscious. Every individual has faced habits they needed to overcome, and more often than not, it is difficult to do something else, make a change in what was always the way such things were done. The literature of the Alexander Technique recognizes that there is a social nature to habit. Observing how babies and toddlers act, one can see that they sit, stand, and move naturally. We can see how toddlers lift objects to their faces instead of slouching over them to see. Toddlers squat down to pick up an object instead of bending over to pick up the object. Habits that contribute to misuse of the body through adulthood come from watching and imitating adults and family members and from social mores taught by parents, schools, and others. Over time, toddlers lose that innate, natural movement ability, developing habits of misuse of the body. These habits are often reinforced by mental habits, including the stress to achieve in school. Jane Heirich notes at least seven characteristics of a habit:

- A habit is composed of a sequence of acts that follows upon some cue. It is a chain reaction of neural events, with responses in all our tissues.
- By its nature, a habit is repetitive behavior, action, or thought.
- Habit feels "right" and comfortable.
- Habit is relatively automatic and largely unconscious.
- As a stereotyped response to doing some activity, a habit is useful for saving time.
- It is a learned behavior—consciously or unconsciously—but once learned, we rarely think about it.
- Habits come into play as we interact with our environment, and not just from within ourselves. (Heirich 2005, 4)

Good habits are worth keeping, but bad habits, those we know are bad for us or learn that they can harm us, are difficult to change because of how deeply ingrained they are through constant, unconscious repetition over a lifetime. The Alexander Technique requires several lessons over time because, as Alexander said, "un-doing" these habits of long–standing takes time and guidance to change. As discussed earlier, Frank Pierce Jones stated, "For the Alexander Technique doesn't teach you something new to do. It teaches you how to bring more practical intelligence into what you are already doing; how to eliminate stereo-typed responses; how to deal with habit and change" (Jones 1997, 2). To grasp this concept is the first step in understanding the basic principles of the Alexander Technique.

THE BASIC PRINCIPLES OF THE ALEXANDER TECHNIQUE

As mentioned above, while the Alexander Technique requires a more in-depth study, including lessons with a certified Alexander teacher, to begin to understand the technique, there are at least five basic principles or concepts that will aid in starting the journey to appreciating the technique to its fullest extent. These basic principles are universally included in virtually every book or resource on the technique. Knowledge of these principles can help develop an understanding, but they alone will not be enough to fully comprehend it. After reading these principles, a more in-depth look at the literature and lessons with a certified teacher will complete the learning process.

The first principle to comprehend has to do with what is known as "the mind-body connection." In Alexander's early days, most people believed that the physical state acted separately, in an automatic way, without one's mind directing the action. Some individuals today may also believe this way. Alexander came to accept that there is a direct connection between how we think and then how our body moves. Overcoming the commonly held belief about this connection, Alexander said, "It is impossible to separate 'mental' from 'physical' process in any form of human activity" (Alexander 1932, 3). This concept informs the methods of teaching the technique. Alexander teachers do not just treat a student's specific ailment. Alexander lessons focus on the mental attitudes, how the student thinks about what he or she is doing, that may be affecting a lower back pain or a hoarse voice; what other areas of tension may be contributing to the pain or ailment; as well as the specific problem the student is most concerned about. Leibowitz recounted a common example that illustrates how the mind-body connection often manifests itself in beginning lessons.

> A beginning pupil comes for an Alexander lesson and is anxious to learn the technique and to do it correctly. The teacher places a hand on the pupil's neck and asks the pupil not to do anything with his muscles, but just to think what the teacher asks him to think. The teacher instructs the pupil to think of releasing his neck to let his head go forward and up. In response, the pupil pulls his head back in an effort to put his head forward. . . . In an effort to get it right, he does exactly the wrong thing. (Leibowitz and Connington 1990, 61)

While the mind-body connection may seem obvious to us today, it is important to accept this fully, for to understand that thinking and physical functioning are coordinated is to accept the ability to harness mental activity to change how we act physically. Heirich calls this coordinated mind-body connection "The Self as a working unity" (Heirich 2005, 8).

The second basic principle to understand concerns what Alexander considered "sensory awareness" and is often spoken of in conjunction with the opposite form, known as "faulty sensory awareness." When Alexander began exploring what was causing his hoarseness on the stage, he spent much time observing himself in mirrors. Though he could see how he stood, moved, and held his head, he was unable to actually feel this. How he thought about his physical sense was affected by how he thought he had always acted. Our physical actions give us sensory feedback, known as kinesthetic or proprioceptive sense, but that sense is faulty to most of us because habit often dictates how we actually read or understand that feedback. Alexander became concerned about what he called his "debauched kinesthesia," where his sense of feedback about movement and posture was not the same as what he observed in the mirrors. Heirich says, "What is comfortable and familiar feels right. Conversely, what is different or unfamiliar feels wrong" (Heirich 2005, 8). People develop habits that, over time become so automatic, they do not realize what could be wrong or what could cause harm from that habit. To do something different often causes resistance because it flies against what one is used to doing, what feels comfortable and familiar. The process of learning the Alexander Technique is a process of learning to overcome the habits of what one is used to doing. In this process, what is taught will feel wrong while old habits are relearned. This is one of the primary reasons hands-on lessons must be taken with a certified teacher over a considerable amount of time.

The third basic principle to understand is that changing habits requires "awareness of the habit," "inhibition," and "mental directions," three concepts within a specific Alexander Technique context. Most Alexander Technique teachers will work with students to develop these three components so that they can achieve "conscious control." As Leibowitz has said, "Conscious control is our tool for carrying out the main objective of the Alexander Technique: to maintain the poise of the head on top of the lengthening spine in movement and rest" (Leibowitz and Connington 1990, 44). In the discussion of the second basic principle, it was noted that habit becomes automatic and something we do not know is happening. We do what feels good and familiar from habit without thinking consciously about it. In order to relearn how we stand, sit, or move in a way that causes unwanted tension, we need to realize what we are doing, what habits are in play, that cause or contribute to these specific actions. If you look at your shoes and notice that the right shoe is much more worn on the outer edge than the left shoe, you understand that you put more weight and step heavier on the edge of your right foot than your left foot, but you do this unconsciously. Try thinking about walking more evenly or with more weight on your left foot, and your early efforts will find you still unconsciously walking more heavily on your right foot, even though you are trying to change. The Alexander Technique works at "awareness of habit" so that you can reprogram those habits that are unconscious, by bringing your body movement into your consciousness. Bringing a habit out to the conscious self may be achieved on one's own, but typically, habits are so ingrained that it is too hard to do so without guidance, such as that provided by an Alexander Technique teacher who is trained to repeatedly direct the student's attention to how their body moves. Being aware of the unwanted habit and actually changing it is another matter. As mentioned earlier, we tend to resist what isn't familiar, what doesn't feel good. Overcoming this resistance to giving up the old habit for a new way of moving or behaving is the next important step in the Alexander Technique. A conscious decision to try to prevent the old way of doing something has to be achieved, and this is what the Alexander Technique calls "inhibition." New students will realize that there is a brief moment, a small window of conscious opportunity, when awareness of the habit is made and the chance to work at changing it happens before habit dominates again how you move and act. Leibowitz says, "Inhibition is not a muscular effort nor is it a passive decision; it is a mental decision to withhold consent from behaving in a particular fashion," and this must happen during that small window of conscious opportunity when awareness of the habit happens (Leibowitz and Connington 1990, 46). Developing this inhibition, a conscious decision to resist what has become so habitual again takes much time and guidance from a trained Alexander teacher. The last of these three concepts, mental directions, is the next step. After learning to resist the old habit, one must direct body movement to behaving in a new way, to learn a new habit, or more precisely, consciously choose to replace the old habit with the directions for behaving in ways that are not a misuse of the body or will not create unwanted tensions. If you discover that you walk too heavily on the side of your right foot, mental directions are those conscious responses you tell yourself to change how you walk on your left and right foot. In the Alexander Technique, the main objective is "to maintain poise of the head on top of the lengthening spine and at rest." To achieve this, there are four common mental directions that are taught in an Alexander Technique process:

1. Allow your neck to release so the head can balance forward and up.
2. Let the torso lengthen and widen.
3. Let the legs release away from the torso.
4. Release your shoulders out to the sides.

These directions, guided by a skilled Alexander Technique teacher and learned over the length of several lessons, will create the ability to control the use of the body and movement, or "conscious control." These three steps, awareness of the habit, inhibition, and mental directions, must work in concert to realize "conscious control."

The fourth basic concept concerns a common obstacle to achieving "conscious control," known as "end-gaining." Most of us are taught that we need to achieve important goals in our life. To do so, we are also taught to work hard to achieve those goals. The goals are ends or results at the end of a process, an education to earn a college degree, a job-hunting process to get a good job, and so forth. We keep our eye on completing the task to get to that goal, and we are often rewarded for achieving it, good grades in school, good salary in employment, and so on, reinforcing the need to reach ends or results in life. This makes us goal oriented in most everything we do. In the Alexander Technique, the focus on achieving the end result is called "end-gaining," and it is considered an obstacle to the process of undoing a habit of misuse of the body. When Alexander observed himself in front of mirrors, his initial thoughts were to find relief for his hoarseness. This was what he wanted to achieve, his end goal. He found that focusing on that end interfered with learning how to become aware of his habit and the process of re-learning it, or undoing it. It is natural for all of us to want to realize our goal, which for many Alexander students is to achieve a life without pain. Many Alexander Technique teachers emphasize that the process of learning to undo old habits must take precedent over getting the result of good, pain-free use of the body.

The fifth basic principle is known as "primary control," sometimes referred to as "primary reflex," a specific concept unique to the Alexander Technique. Alexander used this term to label the relationship of the head to the neck, and the position of the head and neck to the rest of the torso or body. This concept is more than just the position of these body features. It is more important to understand that there is a balanced relationship between the head, neck, and torso, purposeful and compelling to the point of vibrancy as a relationship. Alexander believed that the head, neck, and back have this relationship, and it is important to view it as such rather than each part in juxtaposition with the others, a static poise as Heirich has called it. Primary control is what will be achieved when the four mental directions, described above, are working well. These mental directions must be followed in the order listed for them to work well. In this manner, that relationship between the head, neck, and back or torso will be its most dynamic. Ideally, when primary control is at its optimum, one will move with a minimum of effort. Furthermore, during movement, the back will be supported and the head will be free on top of the neck, and the legs will be able to move freely in the hips.

WHAT HAPPENS IN A TYPICAL ALEXANDER TECHNIQUE LESSON

Most of the Alexander Technique literature, especially journal and magazine articles discussing the technique in general, as well as most websites, feature a discussion on what happens in a typical Alexander Technique lesson. There are common themes or FAQ's in these discussions. The most important are as follows:

1. The number of lessons needed: An exact number cannot be determined because each person is a unique individual with unique issues and learning ability. However, because habits are difficult to undo, a small number of lessons cannot be anticipated. Alexander would work with students for thirty lessons, and the range most often stated is thirty to forty lessons.
2. Frequency of lessons: To work diligently and effectively, it is best to take one or two lessons per week.

3. Length of lessons: Each lesson can be as little as thirty minutes and as long as one hour. Most lessons are in the range of thirty to forty-five minutes. Most Alexander teachers believe that sessions longer than one hour are not very productive.
4. Location of lessons: Typically, Alexander Technique teachers are private practitioners and, therefore, work out of an office or their home studio. Some Alexander teachers work in institutions such as universities, hospitals, pain clinics, and physical therapy clinics.
5. What each student should not expect: Special clothing is not needed, nor do sessions require the student to remove any clothing. Because table work is common in some lessons, women often find it more comfortable to wear slacks or jeans instead of skirts or dresses.
6. What happens in a first lesson: A first session of Alexander Technique lessons is designed to gather information on the student. This usually includes questions about lifestyle, such as where you work and what kinds of activities you do. The teacher is gathering information on how you use your body for sitting, standing, and moving in your normal activities. During this information-gathering phase, the teacher will also observe your posture, how you hold your head, how your back is situated in juncture with your head and neck, and the movement patterns you are using. One of the most important ways the teacher will gather information during this lesson will be with the use of her or his hands. Using gentle touch, the teacher's hands will be placed on the student's neck, shoulder, and back. This aids the teacher's assessment of how you use your body in movement and while at rest. These observations, including the placing of hands on the student's body, will also be performed while the student moves. The teacher will have the student do some simple movements such as walking, sitting, or standing. The first lesson is not all observation. The teacher will also verbally convey information to the student, especially while guiding, through the use of his or her hands, the student's body in movement. This process is designed to begin teaching the student to release their restrictive muscular tension.
7. What happens in subsequent lessons: The additional lessons are designed to work on movement through developing primary control. These sessions are practical in nature and involve hands-on instruction by the teacher while the student moves through a specific task or while the student is lying down, or both. No two teachers approach these lessons alike. There is no standard or set method for each class. Much of the instruction will also depend on the student's needs and ability to develop awareness of habit, inhibition in overcoming that habit, and mental directions to undo and replace unwanted habits with a more desirable means of accomplishing or completing the action at hand. Further lessons may find the teacher addressing how the Alexander Technique can be applied to specific daily activities.

REFERENCES

Alexander, F. Matthias. 1910/1918. *Man's supreme inheritance*. Repr. New York: Dutton.

——. 1923. *Constructive conscious control of the individual*. London: Methuen.

——. 1932. *The use of the self*. New York: Dutton.

——. 1941/1947. *The universal constant in living*. Repr. New York: Dutton.

——. 1995. *Articles and lectures*. Ed. Jean M. O. Fischer. London: Mouritz.

Dart, Raymond A. 1996. *Skill and poise*. Ed. Alexander Murray. London: STAT Books.

Dewey, John. 1939. *The quest for certainty*. New York: G. P. Putnam.

Evans, J. A. 2001. *Frederick Matthias Alexander: A family history*. Chichester, UK: Phillimore & Co.

Garlick, David. 1990. *The lost sixth sense: A medical scientist looks at the Alexander Technique*. Kensington, Australia: Author, University of NSW.

Gelb, Michael. 1981. *Body learning: An introduction to the Alexander Technique*. New York: Delilah Books.

Heirich, Jane Ruby. 2005. *Voice and the Alexander Technique*. Berkeley, Calif.: Mornum Time Press.

Jones, Frank P. 1976. *Body awareness in action: A study of the Alexander Technique*. With a foreword by J. McVicker Hunt. New York: Schocken Books.

——. 1997. *Freedom to change: The development and science of the Alexander Technique*. London: Mouritz.

Kosminsky, Jane, and William Hurt. 1999. *First lesson: An introduction to the Alexander Technique*. VHS. New York: Wellspring Media.

Leibowitz, Judith, and Bill Connington. 1990. *The Alexander Technique*. New York: Harper Perennial.

Rolland, Paul. *The teaching of action in string playing*. Rev. ed. New York: Boosey and Hawkes.

Sanfilippo, Phyllis. 1987. *The Reader's Guide to the Alexander Technique: A Selected Annotated Bibliography*. Long Beach, Calif.: Centerline Press.

1

General Texts and Articles

This chapter includes works that discuss the Alexander Technique in a general nature, especially publications that do not have a specific discipline as its focus. Many of the texts and articles are designed to promote the technique and its basic tenets regardless of what application or discipline that might be applied, as well as the general benefits for anyone who takes training in the method. Some of the works have been written by teachers of the technique, including a few by noted protégés of F. M. Alexander, such as Walter Carrington and Patrick Macdonald. Many of these works describe the training experience a pupil will undergo during Alexander Technique lessons and different aspects of teaching the technique. This chapter includes some biographies of F. M. Alexander and his family, as well as some biographies or testimonials of individuals from different walks of life who benefited greatly from Alexander Technique training. There are a few entries that discuss the spiritual connections and benefits of the Alexander Technique as well. In the "books" section of this chapter, several entries do not include an annotation. These materials were not available through lending libraries, especially those with access through the Online Computer Library Center (OCLC) online database. Most of these publications are from foreign sources and may be available in European or other world libraries. They have been included here to identify them as possible sources useful in learning more about the Alexander Technique.

BOOKS

Arsenault, Michele. *Moving to Learn: A Classroom Guide to Understanding and Using Good Body Mechanics.* **Atlanta, Ga.: Move to Learn Society, 1998.**
Arsenault has developed a textbook on the Alexander Technique that could be used for a course or training workshop. The audience focus of the instruction in the book is children, but it is equally useful for training adults. Arsenault notes that this is a program of learning activities to "actively engage children in a scientific hands-on exploration of human body use potential." These instructions and activities are the product of a pilot project involving almost one hundred children, kindergarten through fifth grade. The children participated in movement activities designed to challenge their body use understanding and in hands-on table lessons during breaks. The activities are most useful for older elementary-aged children, but Arsenault notes that they could be adapted for adults with few alterations. The book is organized into five units: (1) observing ourselves, (2) the body as structure, (3) structure and the forces that act on them, (4) human mechanics and the art of movement, and (5) the balanced body: equilibrium and the efficient use. There are a total of twenty-six lessons, with an average of five activities per unit. Each lesson is composed of an introduction to the topic and a series of from four to six activities. Most of the activities are described in a page or less, many with illustrations. There are several appendixes, including suggested assessments.

Binkley, Goddard. *The Expanding Self: How the Alexander Technique Changed My Life.* **London: STAT Books, 1993.**
Binkley provides his autobiographical account within the context of how the Alexander Technique influenced his life. His story is written in three parts. Part 1 covers his first thirty years of life, which he characterizes as "back trouble, doubt, and depression." This section begins with a narrative of his early life but switches to diary or journal entries in chronological order. In the last entries, he describes how he discovered the Alexander Technique and the Alexander Foundation School. In part 2, Binkley reproduces all of his journal entries of his introduction to Frederick Matthias Alexander and the history of his progress being taught by Alexander, from 1951 to 1953. In his third part, the journal entries continue recording his progress in the training course between 1953 and 1957, under the tutelage of Walter Carrington. Carrington provides a foreword to the book.

Bloch, Michael. F. M.: *The Life of Frederick Matthias Alexander, Founder of the Alexander Technique.* **London: Little, Brown, 2004.**
Bloch, a prolific author of biographies, including several on the Duke and Duchess of Windsor, as well as a noted biography of Count von Ribbentrop, has written a readable yet authoritative biography of F. M. Alexander. He had the support of Walter Carrington, Glynn Macdonald, and Jean Fischer in the preparation of the

manuscript. Fischer aided his work by assisting in obtaining access to a significant number of unpublished letters of F. M. Alexander. The biography is organized into eight chapters: (1) Tasmania (1869–1889), (2) Australia (1889–1904), (3) London (1904–1914), (4) America (1914–1924), (5) Progress (1924–1939), (6) War (1939–1946), (7) Trial (1944–1948), and (8) Finale (1948–1955). The foreword is written by Walter Carrington. There are eight pages of black-and-white photographs of F.M., family members, and pupils.

Bouchard, Ed, and Ben Wright. *Kinesthetic Ventures: Informed by the Work of F. M. Alexander, Stanislavski, Pierce, and Freud.* Edited by Michael Protzel. Chicago: MESA Press, 1997.
The authors, Bouchard, an Alexander Technique teacher, and Wright, a professor of education and psychology at the University of Chicago, found parallels in the study of human consciousness in the works of F. M. Alexander, Konstanine Stanislavski, and Sigmund Freud. Each of these famous men discovered that emotion, body, and mind are incontrovertibly linked. The authors saw other parallels, that all three faced significant resistance to their ideas but overcame them, and "each discovered that learning not to interfere with innate process can transform existence profoundly and that interrupting habitual responses is key." Bouchard and Wright apply Charles Sanders Pierce's semiotic analysis of knowledge and action to clarify and build a greater understanding of Alexander, Stanislavski, and Freud. They argue that "sensory experience, emotion and thought are body learned and body perpetuated." The book contains eleven chapters that integrate the teachings of Alexander into concepts taught by Freud and Stanislavski. For example, chapter 1 describes the relationship and parallels of Alexander's teachings to Freud's concepts of the id, ego, and superego; and chapter 6, entitled "Ah," describes Stanislavski's use of "right imagery to reach pre-verbal back experiences." There is a significant discussion of Charles Sanders Pierce's semiotics, noting that Pierce defined three categories of experience (Firstness, Secondness, and Thirdness) as ways of knowing to account for being and becoming. The final chapter describes the concept of free will as it relates to the teachings of Freud and Alexander.

Brennan, Richard. *Alexander Technique: A Practical Introduction.* Shaftesbury, UK: Element, 1992.
What makes this book by Brennan different from several of his other works is the generous use of step-by-step exercises interspersed throughout each chapter. The text has few illustrations, using a handful of black-and-white drawings, but there is a very thorough explanation of the Alexander Technique, its fundamentals and applications. Beginning with a readable chapter on basic concepts, such as primary control, faulty sensory perception, direction, and inhibition, the remainder of the book has a logical, linear progression through prime topics for learning the Alexander Technique. Starting with a chapter on "how to begin to help ourselves," on awareness and observation, Brennan takes the reader through a chapter by chapter coverage of the mechanics of movement, faulty sensory perception,

inhibition, direction, senses, habits and choices, muscles and reflexes, means and ends, and giving the back a rest. As noted, many practical exercises are used to help instruct the reader in learning each aspect. For example, to demonstrate there is a difference between what we are actually doing and what we think we are doing, or faulty sensory perception, Brennan's exercise instructs the reader to: (1) without looking at the feet, place them nine inches apart pointing, straight ahead and parallel to each other, (2) look at the feet to see if you've achieved the intended position, (3) then, look at the feet as you place them nine inches apart and parallel, and (4) ask yourself, what do they feel like? Brennan also provides a chapter on what to expect in an Alexander Technique lesson and concludes with a number of case histories.

Burge, Paul. *The Matter about Words.* London: STAT Books, 1994.

Callaghan, Michael, and Michal Segal. *The Alexander Technique.* London: Authors, 1994.

Carrington, Walter. *The Act of Living: Talks on the Alexander Technique.* Edited by Jerry Sontag. San Francisco: Mornum Time Press, 1999.
This text follows along the same path of Jerry Sontag's earlier work, *Thinking Aloud* (1994) (see entry below). In this edition, twenty-nine talks that were given by Walter Carrington throughout the years at teacher training lessons and recorded by students have been edited and included. There are no duplicate talks from the *Thinking Aloud* title, though some of the topic is similar. From his "Editor's Note," Sontag indicates that the selection of the talks, out of 150 possible, were chosen based on his assessment of which ones most affected the way he thought about his own use. The text includes a significant "foreword" essay by Tris Roberts, who says of the talks, "Walter Carrington uses his gentle, almost hypnotic, quiet rhetoric to lead aspiring teachers to learn how to cultivate the appropriate mindset in their clients." Carrington also provides a brief preface to the book, and Glynn Macdonald pens the introduction. As with the earlier *Thinking Aloud* volume, these talks were spontaneous at the time they were recorded, often during a reading of F. M. Alexander's books by Carrington, who stopped to expand upon a point extemporaneously. The earliest talk, on spinal curvature, was given in 1988 and, the latest, on "working the wheel," a discussion of the breathing process, given in 1997. Other enlightening talks include (1) habits of thought and action, (2) sciatica, (3) a visual impression, (4) everything flows, (5) yin and yang, (6) gravitation, and (7) change without changing. His final talk included in the text is "the Act of Living," which Sontag says is Carrington's legacy to the world, that is, the point of life is to live life fully.

———. *The Foundation of Human Well-Being: The Work of Professor Magnus and the F. M. Alexander Technique.* London: STAT Books, 1994.

———. *Personally Speaking: Walter Carrington on the F. M. Alexander Technique.* London: Mouritz, 2001.

———. *Thinking Aloud: Talks on Teaching the Alexander Technique.* **Edited by Jerry Sontag. San Francisco: Mornum Time Press, 1994.**

Sontag compiled and edited a significant number of Walter Carrington's talks that were given throughout the world during his teachers' training course or to the Nicholls Training Course in Melbourne, Australia. Many of these talks were recorded by students under his tutelage, so they are edited versions of sometimes spontaneous talks. The earliest talks come from 1966 and span twenty-four years. Organized into twenty-five separate presentations, the talks on the whispered "ah" and on riding are actually the result of several talks combined. Carrington provides a brief preface to the work and said, "I hope that readers will find this little book useful and enjoyable . . . they were given in a casual spontaneous manner without forethought or preparation and certainly without any notion of eventual publication." Some of the more enlightening talks discuss the following: (1) "at our Mother's knee," concerning misdirected energy and sources of energy, (2) lengthening in stature, (3) allowing time to say no, (4) the demand of the constant, (5) the importance of a teacher's use, (6) ethics, (7) nondoing, and (8) taking time. These talks vary in length with most from two to four pages.

———. *A Time to Remember: A Personal Diary of Teaching the F. M. Alexander Technique in 1946.* **London: Sheildrake Press, 1996.**

Chance, Jeremy. *The Alexander Technique.* London: Thorsons, 2001.

Designed as a quick and easy guide to the fundamentals of the Alexander Technique, Jeremy Chance's book is derived from his text *Principles of the Alexander Technique*, published in 1998. This compact, little book is colorfully illustrated with full-page, color photographs throughout. Each concept or term is described in a brief, page-length text, using a more readable font. There is coverage of what the technique consists of and a brief explanation of how F. M. Alexander discovered the technique. The bulk of the text takes one concept or term at a time, using, on average, a half page of text and a full color photograph to illustrate the idea presented. Beginning with what a lesson will entail, the discussion flows from chair work, through table work, and activities. In the section on working on yourself alone, "primary control" is defined and illustrated moving to other concepts, including proprioception, remaining still, self-acceptance, and working seated. The remainder of the text explains concepts and issues of movement, such as working in semisupine position, mapping and releasing, working, standing with mirrors, discovering backwards and down, shortening, and experiencing forwards, forwards and up, and lengthening. Chance also provides a list of useful addresses and websites of Alexander Technique organizations.

Chance, Jeremy. *Thorson's Principles of the Alexander Technique.* London: Thorsons, 1998.

This book is Chance's primary text on the Alexander Technique. Chance was the editor of *Direction*, the journal of the Alexander Technique, for more than fifteen years. After an overview, where Chance likens Alexander lessons to an adventure and excites the reader with the possibilities the technique can realize for an individual, he describes basic physiology of movement, including body movement principles, muscles, motor neurons, and especially inhibitions as freedom. One of the most important chapters regards the anatomy of movement. Here Chance describes the four Alexander directions. He does this with the specific context of body parts: rib cage, lower back, pelvis, and torso and spine. He concentrates on the second direction in these discussions: what you actually think. Another important chapter describes "working on yourself alone," which cautions the reader to work with a teacher to be aware in order to develop conscious habits. He goes on to describe the components of a typical lesson. In a unique chapter on "teaching lineages," Chance provides a brief biography, then explanation, of the teaching styles of three early and prominent teachers of the Alexander Technique: Walter Carrington, Patrick Macdonald, and Marjorie Barstow.

Craze, Richard. *Alexander Technique.* **London: Teach Yourself Books, 1996.**
This practical guide is designed for concise explanations of the Alexander Technique and its applications, but a thorough coverage of all aspects, from history of the technique to how to teach yourself, is an attribute. The book is part of a series of self-help guidebooks in a wide variety of fields, not just the healing arts. Each concept, term, or point is explained in a half page or less. In addition to a coverage of the history of the Alexander Technique and a chapter on the fundamentals, Richard Craze describes what the Alexander Technique is used for and who can benefit from it. Several case studies are employed to introduce who can benefit from the technique, and Craze also describes the typical suitable candidates. Two chapters explain how a teacher would train someone and how one can learn the technique on one's own. Craze promotes the use of charts to record practical exercise applications and track progress. A final chapter describes anatomical issues and concerns, such as the spinal column, head, neck, back, muscles, and nerves. The book is illustrated somewhat sparsely with black-and-white drawings, but they are strategically placed and clearly understood for the concept illustrated.

Dart, Raymond A. *Skill and Poise.* **London: STAT Books, 1996.**
This is a reproduction of most of the centenary collection of writings of Professor Raymond Dart, a South African anatomist who befriended F. M. Alexander in the 1940s and advanced the principles of the technique through his writings. Dart is the creator of the Dart Procedures often included in many Alexander Technique training schools. This work is the brainchild of Alexander Murray, a professor and Alexander Technique teacher who spent several years attempting to get various publishers interested in this compilation. Murray prepared the final essay in the book on "The Dart Procedures." Dart, a respected anthropologist at the time, posited the theory that human evolution has not been a single, progressive string of events and that the evolution of man walking upright was followed by brain expansion. His interests in these areas of evolution and anatomy led him to Alexander and his lessons on the technique in the early 1940s. Six writings of

Dart are included, such as (1) "The Significance of Skill," written in 1934, which discusses the skills Dart considered fundamental to humanity, including erect skills, coordinated eye-hand movement, accurate eye work, mastery of language, and mastery of music; (2) a tribute to F. M. Alexander; (3) voluntary musculature of the human body: the double-spiral arrangement, written in 1950, a treatise on the head-neck relationship; (4) the postural aspect of malocclusion, written in 1946, an essay on posture as it relates to skull and dental abnormalities and issues; (5) the attainment of poise, written in 1947, a treatise on proper posture, including scientific studies and a description of his work with Alexander and in his technique lessons; and (6) weightlessness, written in 1949, a lecture on Feldenkrais's "Body and Mature Behavior." Murray's essay on the Dart Procedures is copiously illustrated with black-and-white diagrams and drawings. An extensive glossary of terms is also included.

de Alcantara, Pedro. *The Alexander Technique: A Skill for Life*. Ramsbury, UK: Crowood Press, 1999.
This tome was written by cellist Pedro deAlcantara, who studied the Alexander Technique under Patrick Macdonald and Shoshana Kaminitz in London, then practiced under the supervision of Wilfred Barlow. This useful text is designed with detailed explanations but with very little in the way of illustrations or photographs. There are six chapters explaining major concepts and applications, and two chapters devoted to the application of the Alexander Technique in (1) sports and exercise and (2) the performing arts. A final chapter is a brief description of the author's experience learning to be an Alexander Technique teacher and how to find one's own teacher. The author provides a thorough explanation of "first principles" in chapter 1, such as the unity of being, causes of misuse, primary control, and sensory awareness and habits. Other chapters discuss "use of the self," "inhibitions and direction," and the essentials of a typical lesson. In one of the more unusual chapters, deAlcantara discusses emotions and the benefits of the Alexander Technique for this concern, in a sensitive and thorough essay. He describes the importance of the unity of body and mind for emotional health and discusses primary emotional phenomena and the application of the Alexander Technique, such as detachment, change, inhibition in the expression of feelings, and issues of personal relations. In one illustrated example, the act of kissing between one partner shorter than the other is described and proscribed. In his discussion on "nondoing," deAlcantara describes how the Alexander Technique gives the ability not to react to a situation, which can be very beneficial in many instances.

deLlosa, Patty. *The Practice of Presence: Five Paths for Daily Life*. Sandpoint, Idaho: Morning Light Press, 2006.

Dimon, Theodore, Jr. *The Undivided Self: The Alexander Technique and the Control of Stress*. Berkeley, Calif.: North Atlantic Books, 1999.
In his foreword to *The Undivided Self*, Walter Carrington states, "(Dimon) treats the concept of the use of the self, not in a restricted sense of the use of the body

and limbs in activity and movement, but comprehensively, including the brain, mind, thought, feeling, and emotion." Theodore Dimon argues that a true concept of mind-body unity requires the identification of underlying causes through a dynamic understanding of the functioning of the mind-body relationship. He found that the articulation of mind-body unity is grounded in the knowledge that the mind and body are a functioning system. Consciousness, then, is not the mere employment of awareness for therapeutic purposes, but rather it is moving from awareness to controlling one's own behavior from within. After an extensive discussion of a unified model of mind and body, Dimon describes the inherent design of the body and then describes how stress must be viewed and analyzed in a complete way. Conventional thinking sees the physical problems of stress caused by mental or emotional responses. The holistic or complete view is to regard physical influences on stress creation as well. To this end, Dimon argues for a conscious process of learning the mind-body unity functioning that affects stress in both physical and mental manifestations. In his appendix, he describes each of the more well-known mind-body techniques, including the Alexander Technique, hypnosis, psychoanalysis, yoga and meditation, massage, and chiropractic.

Dimon, Theodore, and Richard Brown. *Frank Pierce Jones: Collected Writings on the Alexander Technique.* Cambridge, Mass.: Alexander Technique Archives, 1998.

This text is a collection of forty different articles and other published works written by Frank Pierce Jones, one of the world's leading scholars on the Alexander Technique. There is a brief foreword and introduction, the latter written by Dimon, and a ten-page biography of Jones by the authors. Jones was a professor of classical languages at Brown University when he visited A. R. Alexander for lessons to relieve his back pain. After lessons with F. M. Alexander in 1940, Jones was inspired to become a teacher and scholar of the technique. Alexander Murray, in his foreword, asserts for the reader, "The full account of Frank Pierce Jones's quarter of a century of investigations you hold in your hands at this moment." The first article in this work, "Finding the Whole Person," was published as a review of two of Alexander's books (*Man's Supreme Inheritance* and *The Universal Constant in Living*) for the Providence, Rhode Island, newspaper. The last entry in this text, "Head balance as a postural mechanism in man," was submitted to *Science* in 1975 as a response to Niko Tinbergen's Nobel Prize acceptance speech. It was lost in the mail and never published prior to the current text. These entries run the gamut from journal article to newspaper piece to letters to the editor, as well as papers delivered in various educational settings.

Drake, Jonathan. *The Alexander Technique in Everyday Life.* London: Thorsons, 1996.

Most of the chapters of Jonathan Drake's book utilize a lively set of black-and-white photographs of the same model demonstrating the concept being presented. The photographs are often a sequence of photos showing progression of movement or the right position versus the wrong one (marked with an X). In part 1, Drake explains the fundamentals, including "what is good body-use" and "primary control." In "what's good body-use," for instance, he lists two criteria for determining the quality of voluntary movement: (1) absence of effort and (2) reversibility. He also provides a brief history of the technique. In this first part, there is a discussion on "how to change," which describes habitual movement and dealing with inhibition. In the second part, he describes and illustrates eight specific topics in a practical guide, including: (1) the importance of lying down, (2) the head-neck relationship, (3) use of the legs in standing, walking, and running or jogging, (4) sitting and related concerns, (5) lifting, (6) breathing, and (7) specific applications in exercising, swimming, tai chi, and musical performance.

———. *Body Know-How: A Practical Guide to the Use of the Alexander Technique in Everyday Life.* **London: Thorsons, 1991.**
This compact guide provides a layman's view of mastering the Alexander Technique. Illustrated copiously with black-and-white photographs and graphics, the bulk of the text is devoted to very practical exercises and applications. The first three chapters explain the fundamentals in (1) what is good body use, (2) primary control, and (3) how to change. All of these chapters are written for a general audience and are concise readings of no more than four pages per topic. The "primary control" chapter has a very focused discussion, fully illustrated, on the relationship between neck, head, and back and torso. In the chapters with exercises and applications, one is devoted to answering questions, concerns, and misunderstandings. Drake includes an excellent chapter on lying down. After explaining why lying down properly is important, he illustrates arm positions, leg positions, and getting up from the position. One chapter concentrates on the head and its movement and position, while a succeeding chapter is on leg movements (standing, walking, and jogging). These are followed by exercises and descriptions for applying the Alexander Technique while sitting (chapter 8) and lifting (chapter 9). In the discussion on sitting, common sitting activities are explained, including working with chairs, keyboarding, writing, brushing your teeth, reading, and driving. Drake has three very practical appendixes, including (1) ergonomic suggestions, with a discussion of chairs and writing slope, (2) Alexander Technique addresses, and (3) ergonomic and posture aids and products.

———. *Thorson's Introductory Guide to the Alexander Technique.* **London: Thorsons, 1993.**

Evans, J. A. *Frederick Matthias Alexander: A Family History.* **Chichester, UK: Phillimore, 2001.**
This work is the definitive biography of F. M. Alexander, written by his grandnephew, J. A. Evans. Evans uses extensive documentation and interviews with a large number of family members with whom he enjoyed open access as a direct descendent of the Alexander family. He also consulted extensively with prominent

Alexander teachers, Marjory Barlow (also a relative and niece of F. M. Alexander), Margaret Goldie, Erika Whittaker, Walter Carrington, and Elisabeth Walker. F. M. Alexander was the grandson of Matthias Alexander, a hurdle maker banished to Tasmania for his involvement in the Captain Swing Riots of 1830 in England, an agrarian revolt over the growing introduction of the thresher machine. Rural poverty was exacerbated greatly by the loss of jobs when farmers switched harvest production to the thresher. Matthias and his brother John, a carpenter, were sentenced to "transportation" for seven years, a term for banishment to another area of the realm, with Matthias ending up in Stanley, Tasmania. This readable story is divided into four parts: (1) a history of the Alexander family prior to F.M.'s birth, including the account of the Captain Swing Riots; (2) F.M.'s birth and early life, including his career as a "reciter" or pubic speaker, and the earliest developments of his technique; (3) Alexander's career developing and teaching his technique, including his final years; and (4) a tribute to F.M. by John Gray. The book is copiously illustrated with black-and-white photographs, prints, and maps. It also includes an extensive and detailed set of genealogical charts of the Alexander family, beginning with family members born in the early 1700s.

Fischer, Jean M. O., ed. *The Congress Papers: An Ongoing Discovery: Looking towards the 21st Century. From the 6th International Congress on the F. M. Alexander Technique, 9–14 August, 1999, Freiburg, Germany.* London: STAT Books, 2001.

This text reproduces the proceedings of the 6th International Congress on the F. M. Alexander Technique, held in Germany in 1999. The book is organized into two primary sections: (1) Keynote address, topics, evening lectures, and senior guest teachers and (2) Forum: special interest classes. The keynote address was delivered by Tony Spawforth. Walter Carrington's "Alexander and Emotion," written in 1998, is also included in this section. Other evening lectures and senior guest teachers included Mary Cox, Cathy Madden and Jeremy Chance, Lucia Walker and Kevin Martin, Hans Georg Brecklinghaus, Ernst Peter Fischer, and Elisabeth Walker. An interview with Erika Whittaker, conducted by Bruce Fertman, is also reproduced. Topics of these lectures include emotions (Cox), communication (Madden and Chance), concepts (Walker and Martin), and use of the self in ancient Egyptian and classical Greek cultures (Brecklinghaus). Some of the special interest classes included (1) "The Cranio-sacral System" by Hillegonda Boode, (2) "The Primary Control" by Rivka Cohen, (3) "A Turn of Heart" by Bruce Fertman, (4) "Communication and Vocal Use for the Alexander Teacher" by Jane Heirich, (5) "Discovering the Moment of Choice" by John Hunter, (6) "Using the Arms" by Jamie Mc-Dowell, (7) "The Dart Procedures" by Robin Simmons, and thirteen other classes, including the poem "Sun Eclipse" by Carol Levin.

Fischer, Jean M. O. *The Philosopher's Stone: Diaries of Lessons with F. Matthias Alexander.* London: Mouritz, 1998.

Fischer has assembled six artifacts recording experiences with F. Matthias Alexander and his instruction on the Alexander Technique. Four of these artifacts are actual diaries, recorded by dated entry, and written by specific individuals. The first artifact is a reprint of an article originally published in the *Atlantic Monthly*, in April 1919, by Professor James Harvey Robinson, entitled "The Philosopher's Stone." Robinson reminisces about his encounters with Alexander, his book *Man's Supreme Inheritance*, and his experiences learning the technique. The four diaries include those of (1) Eva Webb, who studied with Alexander in 1947; (2) Frank and Grace Hand, from their lessons in 1942; (3) a Miss G.R., published in *Inside Yourself* as "Recording a Miracle" by Louise Morgan in 1954; and (4) Sir George Trevelyan, who worked with Alexander between 1936 and 1938. The final essay is by Anthony Ludovici, originally published in 1961 in *Religions for Infidels*, entitled "How I Came to Have Lessons with F. M. Alexander." Ludovici describes how he became a regular pupil of Alexander in 1925.

Gorman, David. *The Primary Control*. St. Alexandre, France: Learning Methods, 2000.

———. *The Rounder We Go, the Samer We Get*. St. Alexandre, France: Learning Methods, 2000.

———. *Thinking about Thinking about Ourselves*. London: Learning Methods, 2000.

Gray, John. *Your Guide to the Alexander Technique*. New York: St. Martin's Press, 1990.
John Gray, a student and associate of Wilfred and Marjory Barlow, describes the employment of the Alexander Technique, in three sections: (1) Early Lessons, (2) Intermediate Lessons, and (3) Later Lessons. In "Early Lessons," he describes the "Primary Order" and explains and illustrates "neck release," "head forward and up," "back lengthen and widen," and linking Primary Order to experiences. He also describes a working method, including working on a couch and absorbing change, working on oneself, body image (including types of physiques), and general attention and feelings. In "Intermediate Lessons," he explains and describes working through movement, including working with a chair, working against a wall, the "monkey," and hands over the back of a chair. In "Later Lessons," breathing, standing, walking, and working the program are discussed. These discussions are extensive, but a few simple drawings and photos illustrate some of the concepts and activities.

Grennell, Gerard. *Directed Activities: A Diary of Practical Procedures for Students and Teachers of the F. M. Alexander Technique as Taught at the Constructive Learning Centre*. London: Mouritz, 2002.

Hodgkinson, Liz. *The Alexander Technique and How It Can Help You*. London: Judy Piatkus (Publishers), 1988.
In this work, Liz Hodgkinson focuses on how the Alexander Technique benefits an individual physically and emotionally. After a brief explanation of how the technique works, she provides a description of how F. M. Alexander discovered

and developed the technique. She includes a fascinating account of how Alexander influenced Aldous Huxley, who subsequently incorporated the concept into his novels. The main chapters describe the benefits of the Alexander Technique. In the chapter on physical benefits, Hodgkinson provides a thorough discussion of how the Alexander Technique contributes to better health for muscles, back, rheumatism, tennis elbow, and breathing problems. In the chapter on emotional benefits, how the Alexander Technique contributes to mental health, including mental stress, overexertion, Type A personality, and performance anxiety are discussed. Both chapters use a large number of case studies to illustrate key points and issues. Hodgkinson also describes the course of a typical lesson and gives practical exercises for putting the Alexander Technique into one's own practice.

International Alexander Congress. *The Congress Papers: Towards Unity: 2nd International Alexander Congress, Brighton, England, August 1988.* **Bondi, NSW, Australia: Direction, 1988.**
This publication reproduces the speeches and workshops of the 2nd International Alexander Congress, held in Brighton, England, in 1988. The keynote address was by Erika Whittaker, who recounts much of Alexander's life and discusses her perspective of his principles. Michael Frederick addresses the theme of the congress, "Towards Unity," in the first speech. Other prime speeches include David Garlick's "A Physiologist Looks at the Alexander Technique," Sir George Trevelyan's "Act, Don't React," Shmuel Welken's "Postgraduate Study for Alexander Teachers," and Douglass Pierce-Williams's "Loss of Innocence." There are twenty-three workshops included in the Congress papers. Some of these papers are (1) "The Dynamics of Communication" by Lizzie Atkinson, (2) "Acting and Inhibition" by Paul Burge, (3) "The Alexander Technique and Its Application to Back Problems" by Deborah Caplan, (4) "Movement and Voice Improvisation" by Mary Cerny, (5) "Wind Instruments and Respiratory Function," (6) "Present-day Trends in the Upbringing of Children" by Grethe Laub, (7) "We Go Forward and Up" by Glynn Macdonald, (8) "Working with Musicians" by Vivien Mackie, (9) "Applying Chair Work to Cello Playing" by Eckart Richter, (10) "Designing Good Furniture" by Robin Simmons, (11) "Experimental Studies of the F. M. Alexander Technique" by Christopher Stevens, and (12) "Frank Pierce Jones's Views on the Alexander Technique" by Tommy Thompson, and several others.

———. *The Congress Papers: A Spirit of Learning Together: 3rd International Alexander Congress, Engleberg, Switzerland, August 1991.* **Bondi, NSW, Australia: Direction, 1991.**
This publication reproduces the speeches and workshops of the 3rd International Alexander Congress, held in Engleberg, Switzerland, in 1991. The papers are dedicated to Judith Leibowitz, Wilfred Barlow, Patrick Macdonald, and Richard Walker, all who died between the 2nd International Alexander Congress and the 3rd. The keynote address was made by Frank Ottiwell who spoke of the impor-

tance of Alexander Technique professionals coming together periodically to share ideas and to experience a sense of community. Other key addresses include (1) "Our Dancing Motor Units" by Deborah Caplan, (2) "Judith Leibowitz, Her Legacy" by Eleanor Rosenthal, (3) "Good Fences Make Good Neighbors" by John T. Maltsbergen, (4) "Fixation and Fear of Change" by Mary Cox, and (5) "Movement in Context" by Patrick Wall, among others. There are nineteen workshops included in the papers. Some of these are (1) "Running and the Alexander Technique" by Malcolm Balk, (2) "Body Mapping" by William Conable, (3) "In Celebration of the Alexander Technique" by Bruce Fertman, (4) "A Medical Scientist's View" by David Garlick, (5) "Dysfunction in Our Family" by Neal Katz, (6) "Exploring Our Responses in Personal Interactions" by Cathy Madden, (7) "Contact Improvisation" by Lucia Walker, (8) "Let's Get Rid of Group Teaching" by Douglas Wee, (9) "A Matter of Balance" by Douglass Pierce-Williams, and several others.

Macdonald, Glynn. *Illustrated Elements of the Alexander Technique.* London: Element, 2002.

Using colorful photographs and illustrations, the author provides a thorough overview of the Alexander Technique and its applications. Each chapter is directed to the nonpractitioner and describes an important aspect of the technique or a specific application. A brief historical background and biography of Frederick Matthias Alexander begins the book, which includes photos of proper positions and illustrations of the art of breathing. Scientific verification is also described along with an annotated sidebar of Alexander's writings. In the chapter "Use of the Self," the author illustrates breaking habits, conscious inhibition, conscious direction, and sensory application. The photo illustrations colorfully demonstrate each of these discussions. For example, in "breaking habits," a photoset shows a male lifting a box and states, "If I expect the box to be heavy, I make more effort than is necessary." There is a very detailed chapter on anatomy and physiology and a chapter with large photosets illustrating specific procedures, such as walking, lifting, bending, sitting, handwriting, and using a keyboard. Two other chapters discuss and illustrate applications in disciplines. In the chapter for the performing arts, acting, dancing, instrumental music, voice, public speaking, and painting are described, including photo illustrations, and with a case study provided. In the chapter on sports and recreation, riding a horse, bicycling, running, swimming, tennis, golf, skiing, working out, gardening, building and decorating, massage, household chores, and driving a car are also described and illustrated in the same manner. There is also a chapter on the Alexander Technique and medicine.

Macdonald, Patrick. *The Alexander Technique as I See It.* Brighton, UK: Rahula Books, 1989.

Patrick Macdonald, one of the most widely accepted authorities on the Alexander Technique and son of Peter Macdonald, a respected physician and former chair of the British Medical Association, pens his view of the efficacy of the

Alexander Technique. He begins with a "Notebook Jottings" section that is a series of thoughts, ideas, and questions and his comments on those, each beginning "on . . . ," such as "On Trying," "On Effort," and so forth. Most of these entries are a short paragraph of his viewpoint. In his "On Doctors and Drug Houses," Macdonald suggests doctors should rely less on drugs, which he characterizes as "poisons," and more on showing patients how to remove bad habits. He also provides his perspective on F. M. Alexander and his development of the technique and a treatise on "why we learn the technique." In this discussion, he relates the benefits of the Alexander Technique on over ten medical maladies with specific case studies, including asthma, bronchitis, paralysis, torticollis (wryneck), depression, slipped disks, migraine, arthritis, heart trouble, and childbirth. Also included is a description of how to teach the technique that Macdonald argues cogently is both a science and an art. His last chapter reproduces a significant number of testimonials from the famous, including Aldous Huxley and John Dewey, to the medical community.

Macdonald, Robert, and Caro Ness. *Secrets of the Alexander Technique.* London: Dorling-Kindersley, 2000.
This pocket-sized book is fully illustrated with vivid color photographs, designed for a general audience consumption of all the key Alexander Technique concepts, terms, and theory, in an illustrated dictionary-like format. Each concept or term is described and illustrated on no more than two facing pages, with photos dominating the entry. Over one hundred concepts and terms are included, such as the basic concepts of mind-body connection, primary control, identifying habits, sensory appreciation, and conscious inhibition. Entries are grouped into (1) First Steps, where issues of anatomy, movement, and awareness are defined; (2) Teachers in Action, where issues of learning the technique and common everyday activities, such as sitting, reading, writing, driving, breathing, and squatting, among others, are described as to the use of the Alexander Technique; and (3) Self-mastery, describing a variety of life activities including sports, pregnancy and childbirth, emotional support, pain and injury, and working with children.

Massey, Hugh. *An African Odyssey: Evolution, Posture, and the Work of F. M. Alexander: A Memoir.* Bristol, UK: Pomegranate Books, 2001.
Hugh Massey, an anthropologist and engineer, is best known for his study of pygmy societies in the African country of Cameroon. Massey developed the now widely respected theory that evolutionary transition flows from various species of monkeys more than apes and that pygmies are the greater transitional element to the emergence of man. While living among the pygmies of Cameroon during World War II, Massey developed a near fatal case of tuberculosis. Having heard of Alexander's work, Massey underwent instruction on the technique from F. M. Alexander himself. Alexander challenged conventional thinking on the treatment of tuberculosis at the time, which was to reduce activity and breathing. Instead, Alexander believed that full, unimpeded, natural breathing for more efficient and

proper use of the lungs was needed. Massey went into full remission as a result of his Alexander Technique instruction. Additionally, Massey developed the view that evolution is linked to posture in man, which complemented the anthropological work of Raymond Dart. In this text, Massey relates his account of his work in Africa, his bout with tuberculosis and how he was cured by the Alexander Technique, and his subsequent development of his theories that posture plays a significant role in evolutionary history. His account is written in narrative, recounting specific events chronologically in his story. The forward is written by Walter Carrington, who assisted Alexander in his treatment of Massey.

Masterton, Ailsa. *The Alexander Technique in a Nutshell: A Step-by-Step Guide.* London: Element, 2002.
This handy pocket guide to the Alexander Technique is designed for quick and easy reading and understanding of the fundamentals of the technique. Each page is designed and formatted with a full-color photo or graphics, efficient use of white space, and column dividers that compartmentalize text. Most of the components or concepts are explained in two to four pages. Sections include an introduction to the technique and how it was developed, who can benefit from the technique, and why it is an important therapy or procedure. There is an entire section on the mind-body relationship, emphasizing a holistic view. To aid in understanding the technique, concise explanations of habit, stopping to think first, misleading feelings, changing habits, and the relationship of the head, neck, and back are included. In one section, a thorough discussion of muscles and movement is provided and a demonstration of breathing properly. A final chapter provides practical exercises for "helping yourself" in sitting, standing, lying down, writing, and working at a computer.

Maunder, Alex. *Let Your Life Flow: The Physical, Psychological, and Spiritual Benefits of the Alexander Technique.* Essex, UK: C. W. Daniel Co., 2002.
Alex Maunder, trained as an Alexander Technique teacher by Yehuda Kuperman in Basel, Switzerland, writes a very thorough text of the physical, psychological, and spiritual benefits of the Alexander Technique. Half of the book is devoted to the fundamentals of the Alexander Technique, especially what Maunder terms "the tyranny of habits" and the basics of balance, breathing, directions, mental calmness, and primary control. There is also coverage of the history of the technique. Four final chapters address Maunder's focus of the psychological and spiritual benefits. In "the psychological significance of posture," he shows how the Alexander Technique helps the individual peel off layers (using the onion as an analogy) of habits and patterns, but more so, the Alexander Technique shows people the core of our being is the flow carrying the person physically, mentally, and emotionally. Also, the Alexander Technique helps people develop their own "rescue remedy," an inner transformation. In his "psycho-physical rebalancing," Maunder argues that the Alexander Technique is a way of changing habits but

emphasizes that these habits are not just physical but mental and emotional as well. Rebalancing is the way individuals are taught to create a unity of mind and body by relearning these habits. Finally, in his chapter on spiritual benefits, Maunder states, "The purpose of practicing the Alexander Technique may be summed up as a means of focusing and becoming conscious of our true centre, enabling us to identify fully and willingly with that equipoise which is absolute stillness, and from which the extraordinary dynamic of polarity issues as effect." Maunder argues that, because we still have a physical presence, driven by our habits, the answer is "in ceasing to strive to be anything; that we do not exist separately from God, life, the flow—call it what you will—and that the 'personality,' limited by body and matter, needs merely to undergo a shift of identity. We are the flow."

McCaffry, Annie. *Journey to Myself: The Healing Relationships and the Transformation of Family Patterns.* **Shaftesbury, UK: Element, 1992.**
An autobiography of the author's life, Annie McCaffry emphasizes conscious learning of unity of mind and body in overcoming personal, emotional, and physical tragedies and problems. McCaffry's focus is more rooted in the Feldenkrais Method, which dominates her discussion of the therapeutic paths she has explored in overcoming the difficulties from her own family and relationship background, but briefly discusses her meeting Ilana Rubenfeld and learning the Alexander Technique and its benefits. McCaffry suffered with back ailments most of her life and also describes her personal and emotional trials (marriage and divorce, for example) in the first part of the book. McCaffry sought a number of therapists, most notably Feldenkrais, Paul Solomon, and Irene Tasker. In her chapter "Awakening to Disease Where It Is Held in the Body," her commentary is very aligned with the principles of the Alexander Technique, though she rarely mentions it.

McGowan, Daniel. *Constructive Awareness: Alexander Technique and the Spiritual Quest.* **Burdett, N.Y.: Larson Publications, 1997.**
Daniel McGowan views the "scheme of life" as a continuum drawn as a chart to explain the interconnections to a holistic view of life. McGowan relies heavily on the works of philosopher Paul Brunton for this "scheme." At the top of the chart is the "mind," or the "Great Void," likened to the biblical "darkness upon the face of the deep," that which is beyond human thought and imagination. Below this on the chart is "world-mind," which McGowan characterizes as "mind-in-action" and, in religious perspective, God as universal intelligence and creative power. This is then followed by "overself," which is the essence or soul of the individual human being, which is linked to the "World-Mind." McGowan views these first three aspects of the scheme of life as a manifestation of how the universe can be fathomed, from that which cannot be understood through the concept of creation and action, to fundamental consciousness of being. The scheme of life chart then illustrates five components that are the essence of individual being: (1) ego (or reflected conscious-

ness), (2) body, (3) the senses, (4) the environment, and (5) the physical (that which can be touched). For McGowan, the Alexander Technique provides the ability to be consciously aware of these five components of the individual, especially ego, body, the senses, and the environment. His text walks the reader through this understanding, as can be learned by the Alexander Technique, of conscious awareness. He devotes full chapters to an understanding of the body, the power of habit and inhibition, and direction, as fundamentals of the technique. He also describes the benefits of meditation, hatha yoga, and breathing, within this context of conscious awareness and the Alexander Technique. McGowan makes an impassioned argument that the Alexander Technique is not to be viewed as an alternative therapy or health remedy nor as "body work" but rather as a reeducation in the use of the self, based on intelligent reasoning and inspired intellectual analysis.

————. *Going Mental.* Totnes, UK: D. McGowan, 2000.

McLeod, Rosslyn. *Up from Down Under: The Australian Origins of Frederick Matthias Alexander and the Alexander Technique.* Victoria, Australia: Rosslyn McLeod, 1994.
Rosslyn McLeod, a musician and Alexander Technique teacher, has penned a biography of F. M. Alexander's early years. Her work has been informed greatly by access to the correspondence between Alexander and Dr. Alexander Leeper, First Warden of Trinity College, Melbourne. Leeper was an early supporter of Alexander and his technique who advocated for its inclusion as physical instruction in Australian schools. This work includes significant historical detail on early Australia, the history of the Alexander family in England, history and culture of Australia, New Zealand, and Tasmania of the 1800s, and especially the city of Melbourne during Alexander's work there in the 1880s and 1890s. Much of the biography is peppered with actual excerpts of letters, news accounts of the time, and quotes from other publications. About one-third of the book is devoted to a historical account of Alexander's career as an elocutionist and actor leading up to his problems with a faltering voice and his self-discovery process. The final chapters describe his early teaching experiences, especially in Melbourne and Sydney. One full chapter is devoted to his association with Lilian Twycross, a singing teacher and contralto singer, an early student of Alexander's. Another full chapter describes Alexander's association with Leeper. The book includes numerous black-and-white photographs of Alexander, Twycross, Leeper, and Australia of that era.

Murray, Joan, and Alexander Murray, in conversation with Kevin Ahern and Marian Goldberg. *Beginning from the Beginning: The Growth of Understanding and Skill.* Edited by Marian Goldberg. McLean, Va.: Alexander Technique Center of Washington, D.C., 1996.
This work is divided into two distinct sections. Section 1 includes the dialogue of a conversation between Joan and Alex Murray, two well-known Alexander Technique teachers who studied with Walter Carrington and others in the 1950s and

1960s, and Kevin Ahern and Marian Goldberg of the Alexander Technique Center of Washington, D.C. In section 2, full-page, black-and-white photosets illustrate nineteen Dart procedures, particularly emphasizing the natural posture of babies and children. Alex Murray is the inventor of the Murray Flute and is a professor of flute at the University of Illinois as well as the author of numerous articles on the Alexander Technique. The thirteen conversations in section 1 average four pages in length and include topics on early development of the Dart procedures, the Alexander Technique, Dart and the flute, stages of development in teaching, "forward to the beginning: fetal" (a discussion of fetal lengthening), static mysteries or growth (a discussion of novice Alexander Technique teachers' challenges), the double-spiral, creeping, rotating and bipedaling, and a final discussion on "process versus product," a commentary by Alex Murray comparing Dart and Alexander's way of describing the technique.

Oppenheimer, Anne, ed. *The Congress Papers: Exploring the Principles: From the 7th International Congress of the F. M. Alexander Technique, 16–22 August, 2004, Oxford, England.* London: STAT Books, 2005.
This work reproduces the conference proceedings of the 7th International Congress of the F. M. Alexander Technique, held in Oxford, England, in 2004. There are forty-nine papers included in this volume under a conference theme of "Exploring the Principles." Some of the papers include (1) "Group Teaching" by Meade Andrews; (2) "Detached Observations" by John Brown; (3) "Back in the Beginning" by Walter Carrington; (4) "A Tale of Two Paradigms" by Jeremy Chance; (5) "Living without Proprioception and Touch" by Jonathan Cole; (6) "Alexander and Voice Work" by Janet Madelle Feindel; (7) "Decoding Dancerspeak" by Robin Gilmore; (8) "Integrating Eyes, Brain, and Body" by Peter Grunwald; (9) "Golfing with the Alexander Technique" by Martyn Jones; (10) "Teaching without Touching" by Catherine Kettrick; (11) "The Ambush of Fear" by Elizabeth Langford; (12) "Personality Adaptations and the Alexander Technique" by Jamie McDowell; (13) "The Alexander Technique in Pregnancy and Childbirth" by Ilana Machover; (14) "The Whispered 'Ah' and the Expression of Emotion" by Robin Mockli; (15) "What Is Presence on Stage?" by Penny O'Connor; (16) "Thought Shepherding in Singing" by Patricia O'Neill; (17) "Working with the Chakras, Emotions, and the Alexander Technique" by Glen Park; (18) "Teaching the Alexander Technique to People with Parkinson's" by Chloe Stallibrass; (19) "Feet—The Final Frontier" by Jane Staggs, and a panel presentation on neuroscience and the Alexander Technique.

Park, Glen. *The Art of Changing: A New Approach to the Alexander Technique.* Bath, UK: Ashgrove Press, 1989.

———. *A New Approach to the Alexander Technique: Moving toward a More Balanced Expression of the Whole Self.* Freedom, Calif.: Crossing Press, 1998.
Glen Park, a trained Alexander Technique teacher and professional actor, became an ardent Alexander Technique proponent after coming to training for a chronic

back condition. Park has designed a text that can be characterized as two books in one. In the first part, "Fundamentals," Park explains the technique in thorough detail through ten chapters. Contrary to many texts on the Alexander Technique, she does not dedicate a whole chapter to the history of the Alexander Technique but rather includes a short biography of F. M. Alexander as an appendix. Beginning with a chapter on "the use of the self," which is a discourse on observing one's body and habits to discover issues of habitual use, she spends considerable time explaining (1) the semisupine habit, (2) sensory awareness, and (3) how muscles work. Each of these chapters use detailed explanations of the concepts of the Alexander Technique and are illustrated with black-and-white graphics. In her chapter on "primary freedom," the basic concepts of primary control are discussed. She includes a good discussion of "experiencing the weight of the head" and the startle response. One of her best chapters describes "thinking in activity," or working with one's ability to bring about changes through direction. In her chapter "Interfering," she states that the Alexander Technique "offers a return to grace, a coordinated organism, with a reliable sensory mechanism and an advance to conscious control." In the second part of the book, "Developments," Park steps away from Alexander to some degree. She notes that "Alexander seemed to believe that by improving the primary control of a person . . . all emotional and nervous problems would eventually disappear. Unfortunately, this encourages confusion between 'inhibition' as Alexander used the word, and 'inhibition' in the repressive sense that Freud used it." Park designs this second part to address a means of making the technique one's own by looking at other ways of thinking. She includes a chapter on "the emotional body" that examines habitual emotional responses and a chapter on the "thinking body" that combines the Alexander Technique instruction on conscious awareness with issues of emotional response. She also describes the dance of the Shiva and the chakras and relevant parallels to the Alexander Technique.

Robb, Fiona. *Not to "Do": An Account of Lessons in the Alexander Technique with Margaret Goldie, July 1995 to November 1996.* London: Camon Press, 1999.

Roth, Nancy. *Spiritual Exercises: Joining Body and Spirit in Prayer.* New York: Seabury Books, 2005.
Nancy Roth's background and life story, grounded in ballet, has led her to explore the integration of spirituality and body work. She begins by relating three vignettes that demonstrate how this has evolved in her life. In her introduction to the body-work techniques she describes, she makes a cogent argument that prayer and "body spirit" go hand in hand. As she states, "If we are a bodyspirit, and if God is with us in all things, that means that physical exercise can be an integral part of our recollection and prayer." The remainder of the book has two distinct parts: (1) a description of numerous body-work techniques and activities, discussed within a context of spirituality, with specific exercises as suggested value-added experiences, and (2) development of a spiritual life through the integration

of prayer and exercise. In the body-work section, she describes nine techniques and activities, including the Alexander Technique, hatha yoga, tai chi, Pilates, strength training, aerobic exercise, dance, breathing, and walking. In the essay on the Alexander Technique, she provides a brief history of the technique's development and discusses the basic principles. She makes the case that the Alexander Technique teaches us to be good stewards of our body. She includes an exercise with specific, detailed instructions that begin having one sit in a chair, turn the head slowly to look left, then right. Follow this by tipping the head back to look up at the ceiling, then down to the floor. The second section, "Praying through the Body," describes three forms of prayer and how to integrate body work into the process of prayer, including (1) contemplative prayer, (2) reflective prayer, and (3) verbal prayer.

Russell, Mike. *Alexander Technique*. London: Caxton Editions, 2002.
Mike Russell has designed a unique, colorfully illustrated book of the fundamentals of the Alexander Technique using a simple, outlined form for explanations. A first chapter, "Where It All Started," is written in a lively, but simplistic style for the average reader, complete with beautiful color photos drawing the readers' interest to the point illustrated. When a major concept is then introduced, such as "primary control," the explanation is broken down into numbered steps of brief paragraphs, compartmentalizing each aspect of the explanation. Illustrations accompanying each explanation include color photos and graphics. Russell also uses a unique design by programming a "take a break" section between major sections. Each "take a break" section interjects a separate concept that instructs the reader to pull back from the more involved, previous explanation. This "take a break" concept is a significant one but requires less to grasp than the more difficult ones of the major sections where the "take a break" section is embedded, such as "The Monkey" in "Take a Break 2" and "Taking Exercise" in "Take a Break 3." Major sections cover (1) primary control, (2) a day with the Alexander Technique indoors, (3) a day with the Alexander Technique out and about, and (4) more activities indoors (e.g., sewing, ironing, vacuuming, and bathing).

Scarano, Jim. *The Alexander Technique in Daily Life*. Meadowbank, Australia: Random House International, 1997.

———. *The Alexander Technique in the New Age*. Meadowbank, Australia: Random House International, 2000.

Schapera, Vivien Singer. *Everyday Magic*. Cincinnati, Ohio: Four Winds Academy Press, 2002.
Written as a memoir, this autobiography of Vivien Singer Schapera tells her complete story, from birth to the present, and the influences in her life and the many milestones in her development as a healing artist. Most of the text discusses specific events in her life and her explanations of these events. Schapera is the

founder of Four Winds Academy, a healing arts college and a trained and qualified teacher of the Alexander Technique, crystal healing, past-life regression, and medical intuition. As the back cover states,

> The author provides us with the launch points to further study of a variety of disciplines that she has integrated into a seamless and coherent whole. With the Alexander Technique at the core, Schapera shares her discoveries about nutrition, crystals, healing shamanism and other paths, and shows us how they all, in the end, share a common message: magic is within your reach and mine, everyday.

Her beginnings with the Alexander Technique are found midmemoir and are interwoven into her remaining life's story.

Soar, Tim. *Defining the Alexander Technique.* **London: Author, 1999.**

Staring, Jeroen. *The First 43 Years of the Life of F. Matthias Alexander.* **Nijmegen, The Netherlands: Author, 1997.**
This two-volume set is a substantial biography of F. M. Alexander from his birth in 1869 through the production of his book *Conscious Control in Relation to Human Evolution in Civilization*, published in 1912. This work is a limited edition with only fifty copies published. It includes a foreword by Rodney Mace in the first volume and Ed Bouchard in the second volume. The text utilizes a substantial amount of primary source material and quotes extensively from these sources, sometimes at length, throughout the two volumes. The high level of scholarly research is clearly evident. Only the first chapter of volume 1 describes his early years prior to his discovery. The remainder of the two volumes documents his work on the technique. Volume 1 describes how Alexander discovered his technique and then his move to London. There is a substantial chapter on his London writings. Volume 1 ends with an account of Alexander's relationship with Scanes Spicer, a Darwinist who proposed a different theory of the physiology of the mechanism of respiration, and a controversy over Alexander's charge of plagiarism against Spicer. Volume 2 begins with a substantial coverage of "the whispered 'ah'" principle, and the remaining work of this volume is devoted to a significant, documented discussion of three of Alexander's publications, (1) his pamphlet *Introduction to a New Method of Respiratory Re-education*, and his books (2) *Man's Supreme Inheritance*, and (3) *Conscious Control*. Both volumes include an extensive literature collection.

Stevens, Chris. *Alexander Technique: An Introductory Guide to the Technique and Its Benefits.* **London: Vermilion, 1987.**
Chris Stevens, who studied with Walter Carrington, provides a thorough overview of the Alexander Technique and how it can aid one's health. In the first couple of chapters, he explains the fundamentals of what the technique consists of and why it is needed. The author begins with quotes from several well-known people, such as

Monty Python's John Cleese, the author Aldous Huxley, and the playwright George Bernard Shaw, on the value of the Alexander Technique. He includes humorous cartoons to emphasize a point throughout the book. Stevens designs one chapter as an FAQ to many of the common questions about the technique. There is also an excellent chapter with a detailed explanation of four stages of learning, concluding with a description of why the technique takes long to learn, due to the time involved in learning about "self" rather than mind and body. Stevens also provides an excellent description of the scientific evidence supporting the Alexander Technique. He concludes the work with a robust discussion about learning to help oneself.

Stolmack, Margaret. *Coach Yourself.* Milsons Point, Australia: Random House International, 2000.

Taylor, Anthony James. *Whatever You Are Doing Now, You Can Do It Better: Your Guide to the Alexander Technique.* Surrey, UK: Gil Books, 2004. Anthony Taylor provides insight into his teachings within his Alexander Technique course by preparing a text replete with personal anecdotes, quotations from prominent inspirational speakers and writers, and unique analogies that illustrate key concepts. Taylor promotes the view that everyone can improve their life, and he features Steven Covey's *Seven Habits of Highly Effective People* as a complementary guide to his discussion of how the Alexander Technique can improve what anyone does. He includes a full chapter devoted to F. M. Alexander and the history of the technique. This is followed by ten separate chapters, each a core principle of the Alexander Technique, including (1) use of reason, (2) psychophysical unity, (3) prevention, (4) taking simple, manageable steps, (5) mistaking effects for causes, (6) unreliable feelings, (7) fixed, preconceived ideas, (8) mental discipline, (9) genuine trust, and (10) working to principle. Each of these chapters are structured with what Taylor includes in his introductory Alexander Technique course. He also includes an appendix with contact information for Alexander Technique organizations and a brief bibliography.

Weed, Donald. *What You Think Is What You Get: An Introductory Textbook for the Study of the Alexander Technique.* Bristol, UK: Groups in Learning, 1999.

ARTICLES

Cranz, Galen. "The Alexander Technique in the World of Design: Posture and the Common Chair; Part 1: The Chair as Health Hazard." *Journal of Bodywork and Movement Therapies* 4, no. 2 (April 2000): 90–98. The author critiques the Western tradition of chair sitting and chair design, and argues that chair design is based on weak physiological and kinesthetic theory or concepts. He discusses better ways of sitting for posture and health, especially with a detailed discussion of the Alexander Technique. He summarizes the five principles of the Alexander Technique contextually within this discussion of poor chair design. A brief history of chair design follows as a means of answering why the chair and its design has become so important for posture and health. The author concludes that chair designers and users have overemphasized the importance of representing social status in chair designs. In part 2, Cranz develops recommendations for body-conscious furniture and interiors.

Davis, Carol Anne. "Hold Your Head Up: The Alexander Technique." ***Spare Rib*** **192 (July 1988): 50–51.**
In narrative form, the author describes why she sought an Alexander Technique teacher and how her lessons progressed. She begins by recounting her childhood problem of her father constantly snapping at her to walk the way he expected her to do. She sought an Alexander Technique teacher as an adult, and freelance writer, for back pain, assuming her only problem was a stooped back posture. Her first lesson is described in some detail and shows how she learned of her misuse and the Alexander Technique teacher's approach. The author notes that she was walking properly after ten to twelve lessons. A description of the history and development of the Alexander Technique is also provided.

Gilmore, Robin. "Learning to Touch: Contact and Alexander Training in Japan." ***Contact Quarterly*** **20 (Summer/Fall 1995): 65–66.**
Robin Gilmore, director of the Kyoto Alexander Program Promoting Awareness (KAPPA) in Japan, begins by noting that the Alexander Technique requires hands-on instruction in order for the teacher to see overall patterns of muscular use. However, hands-on contact presents cultural issues to overcome in Japan. Another concern comes from the way the Japanese approach educational opportunities so intensely, causing concern for constructive learning. The Japanese custom of bowing with gaze lowered causes a downward pull of the head and neck. Gilmore introduced contact improvisation, using a finger to finger contact, as well as Bartenieff fundamentals. She reports great success in creating enthusiasm and flexibility in her Japanese students.

———. "Moving beyond Fight or Flight." Unpublished manuscript, 2001.
Gilmore notes that most people react with a "fight or flight" response in startling situations. In the context of the Alexander Technique, there is a tightening of muscles and an overall contraction of the body, usually with a gasping of air. Gilmore argues that this is evidence of a mind-body connection. After a brief discussion of the fundamentals of the Alexander Technique, she makes a strong case for employing the Alexander Technique to build a better response to startling news and events. Written after the terrorist attack of September 11, she often mentions the heightened sense of fight or flight events since this tragedy. Gilmore describes an exercise as an example of how the Alexander Technique can be beneficial in these situations.

Household, Nicki. "The Evening Class, Alexander Technique: Mind and Body." *Times Educational Supplement,* **no. 4344 (October 1, 1999, Supp. Friday): 19.**
The author describes the step-by-step events in one Alexander Technique session. She begins by describing the objects used in the class, including several lengths of string, a pile of paperbacks, and a miniature model of a skull. The technique is described as a one-on-one, hands-on method of monitoring the student's posture. The training is designed to implement tiny changes that will eradicate tension.

Johnson, Bonnie. "Judith Leibowitz Teaches Students How to Stand Up and Be Counted Healthy." *People Weekly* **20 (October 17, 1983): 67–68.**
This is a popular magazine biography of famed Alexander Technique teacher Judith Leibowitz. The article reveals her story of contracting polio at a young age and the years of fear while growing up of not being able to walk normally. Leibowitz needed a cane during these years and walked with a limp through her college years. While working as a chemist, she began taking Alexander Technique lessons with Alma Frank. This experience was the impetus to become an Alexander Technique teacher. Leibowitz tells the author her philosophy and method for teaching the technique. Her students have included actors Kevin Kline, William Hurt, and Patti Lupone.

Keresey, Maggie. "Stay Limber Longer: Here's How to Keep the Spring in Your Step for Years to Come." *New Choices* **38, no. 4 (May 1998): 32–36.**
The author makes a commonsense argument that individuals need to choose a consistent exercise and fitness program that fits one's own criteria and lifestyle. She then goes on to describe six programs worth considering for health and fitness, including the Alexander Technique, ballet exercise, yoga, Pilates, tai chi, and the Feldenkrais. Each of the six program descriptions is formatted with six questions, answered briefly, including what it is, how it works, what you wear, benefits, drawbacks, and cost. Alexander Technique benefits listed include improving coordination and flexibility, and drawbacks listed include that practitioners are concentrated in more populous urban areas and may be hard to locate.

Maren, Michael. "Why I'm a Stand-up Guy." *GQ* **64 (March 1996): 64.**
In a popular men's magazine, the author describes his experiences taking Alexander Technique instruction at the Mid-Town Center for the Alexander Technique in New York. Michael Maren explains that he learns that the technique is not about learning to do something different but rather about undoing bad physical habits. He explains that the lessons are not something you can learn from a home video but that it is a hands-on technique. He also found that clinical studies show that the Alexander Technique improves respiratory function.

Moe Glasnow, Debra. "Alexander Technique: Internal Feedback for Reducing Tension." *Let's Live* **62, no. 9 (September 1994): 42–43.**
The author provides a brief overview of the Alexander Technique, including some statistics on the number of teachers and schools worldwide. She also briefly de-

scribes her personal experience with a lesson. A separate sidebar explains the origins of the Alexander Technique and a brief biography of F. Matthias Alexander. Another sidebar gives instructions on locating an instructor.

Morrow, Felix. "William James and John Dewey on Consciousness: Suppressed Writings." *Journal of Humanistic Psychology* **24, no. 1 (Winter 1984): 69–79.**
This article reproduces Felix Morrow's remarks at the 1982 International Conferences convened by the Institute of Noetic Sciences, formed to discuss the means for introducing knowledge of the scope of consciousness into educational systems. The primary focus of the article is to show the evidence of suppression of the writings of William James on psychical research and the concept of cosmic consciousness, and the suppression of John Dewey's works on the integration of the Alexander Technique principle into the educational systems. Morrow found that the literary authorities publishing Dewey's works systematically excluded all of his writings on Alexander and his technique. He meticulously documents the scholarly evidence to show that this occurred. Dewey argued that the Alexander Technique was a model of learning by doing. Dewey believed that Alexander had the best grasp of evolutionary changes in human nature. Dewey also believed that resistance to the Alexander Technique was due to man's fear of the human body. Morrow describes Dewey's thoughts on the Alexander Technique in depth and recounts the forces that opposed him.

Wolf, Francesa. "Get 'em Young and They're Upright for Life." *Times Educational Supplement,* **no. 4089 (November 11, 1994): supp. 5.**
Francesa Wolf describes the efforts of a small number of projects to bring Alexander Technique lessons into the schools. These initiatives all take place in British school settings. She notes that though the Alexander Technique is normally seen as applicable to adults, it is clearly valuable to children as well. One Alexander Technique team instructor in a school in Redhill, UK, observed that nursery children used their bodies in a natural way but saw this disappear in children aged seven and up. Wolf describes the individual accounts of these projects and teams. For example, one team member observed that, during writing lessons, children had their heads down on their desks, with mouths close to their fingers, viewing this as a whole process of contraction. One instructor used "body thinking" in her Alexander Technique lessons with children, using phrases like "I let my neck be free," and others to help them keep the relationship between neck and head. There is a brief description of a typical lesson.

Wolf, Jessica. "The Alexander Technique." In *Selected Breathing Masterclasses.* **Malibu, Calif.: Windplayer Publications, 2002.**

2

Resources for the Performing Arts, Especially Dance, Music, and Theater

The Alexander Technique has been more widely known amongst the professions in the performing arts than in any other field. This is a direct result of F. M. Alexander's professional prospective and his development of the technique as a Shakespearean reciter. Early students of Alexander did come from other disciplines, but the performing arts remained dominant in the dissemination of the technique's use and influence for years. The resources listed below present works from the three main performing arts that have extensive publications on the application of the Alexander Technique for their discipline: music, theater, and dance. Most of these resources are scholarly publications. There are only a few resources from general or popular publications, primarily magazines. The resources for musicians are more often for a specific discipline within music, such as voice or a particular type of instrument. Resources for the theater always address acting ability and skills, which on some occasions includes singing in the musical theater. Resources for dance are general in nature, and not focused on a specific style of dance. In the "books" section of this chapter, several entries do not include an annotation. These materials were not available through lending libraries, especially those with access through the Online Computer Library Center (OCLC) online database. Most of these publications are from foreign sources and may be available in European or other world libraries. They have been included here to identify them as possible sources useful in learning more about the Alexander Technique.

27

BOOKS

Conable, Barbara, and Benjamin Conable. *Course Material for What Every Musician Needs to Know about the Body.* **Portland, Oreg.: Andover Educators, 2001.**

Dimon, Ted. *Alexander Technique and the Voice: Understanding the Whispered "Ah."* **N.p.: Day Street Press, 1996.**
Ted Dimon's text is a concise guide to the Alexander Technique concept of the whispered "ah." A significant amount of information is packed into less than twenty pages of text. There are four sections, two describing and discussing breathing and the voice, and two describing and discussing the whispered "ah." Dimon explains how and why we breathe, noting much of the movement of breathing is not voluntary. He also explains the close relation of breathing to free movement of ribs and diaphragm. In another chapter, Dimon provides an in-depth explanation of how we produce sound and vocal use, and its effect on breathing. In the sections on the whispered "ah," Dimon first defines the elements of this concept by breaking it down into manageable components. He begins with a description of the instructions for the face and throat. A description of "controlled exhalation" is the next component. Dimon summarizes the components as follows: (1) commanding the coordinations, ensuring full and free breathing, (2) breaking the whispered "ah" into the components of facial and throat directions and forms of controlled exhalation, (3) learning to perform a controlled exhalation based on preventing the need to take breath, and (4) paying attention to the "ah" sound. Dimon concludes with a discussion of the whispered "ah" and vocalizing.

Gilmore, Robin. *What Every Dancer Needs to Know about the Body: A Workbook of Body Mapping and the Alexander Technique.* **Portland, Oreg.: Andover Press, 2005.**

Gorman, David. *Working with a Violinist.* **St. Alexandre, France: Learning Methods, 1999.**

Heirich, Jane Ruby. *Voice and the Alexander Technique.* **Berkeley, Calif.: Mornum Time Press, 2005.**
Jane Heirich develops a substantial explanation of the integration of the Alexander Technique in voice instruction and skill development. She begins with a brief discussion of habit and vocal use, the difficulty of changing habit, and the social nature of habit. One chapter is dedicated to the history of the Alexander Technique and its development, but Heirich also provides relevant, practical connections to her discussion of voice training with a description of specific skills learned through the study of the technique. Two chapters follow to discuss fundamentals of voice and the problems poor posture brings to vocal

performance. The remaining chapters are designed as "games and explorations," practical exercises demonstrating specific Alexander Technique and vocal instruction. Chapter 5 describes the reeducation of breathing habits. Chapter 6 takes up the change process. The "monkey" and how it applies to voice training, including exercises, follows in chapter 7. A final chapter covers exercises for supporting the voice. The text is fully illustrated with clear, engaging, black-and-white drawings and diagrams. Several useful appendixes are included, such as the International Phonetic Alphabet, contact information, and notation, pitch name, and frequency correlation chart. The text comes with an instructional CD as well.

Macdonald, Robert. *The Use of the Voice: Sensory Appreciation, Posture, Vocal Functioning, and Shakespearean Text Performance.* **London: Macdonald Media, 1997.**

Robert Macdonald conducted research on the relationship between improvements in sensory appreciation and respiratory and vocal functioning made possible by using the Alexander Technique with three actors performing with specific Shakespearean text from *Richard III, Henry IV*, part 1, and *Hamlet*. Macdonald conducted the research as a case study using these readings of the vocal performance, diaries kept by the participants, including that of Macdonald as practitioner, and a questionnaire completed by the participants upon conclusion of the study. Macdonald developed a series of postural and performance assessments to determine the reliability of sensory appreciation from the data gathered, including (1) increasing recognition of interference with the postural mechanisms, (2) accelerating responsiveness to the manual stimulus given by the teacher, (3) increased awareness of the reflex nature of breathing and voice, (4) ability to operate at full stature while vocalizing, (5) less nervous reaction in performance, and several more similar criteria. Macdonald found, in his analysis of the data that he gathered, that there was a strong association between a low standard of sensory appreciation, poor performance, and vocal functioning, and that at least two of the participants made significant improvements in sensory appreciation and posture after training with the Alexander Technique. Macdonald also includes a chapter in which he discusses the texts of four vocal teachers for their descriptions of the role in posture and sensory appreciation, including the work of Cicely Bernan, Kristin Linklater, Patsy Ralenburg, and Clifford Turner.

Mackie, Vivien, in conversation with Joe Armstrong. *Just Play Naturally.* **N.p.: Duende Editions, 2002.**

Designed as an interview with formatted questions and responses, this work provides an autobiographical account of Vivien Mackie's cello training with Pablo Casals. Joe Armstrong, an Alexander Teacher and student of Mackie, asks the questions. First, Mackie found that Casals's style of teaching cello was largely contrary to her own years of training. Then, after studying for three years with Casals, she began to link lessons from the Alexander Technique that reinforced what she had learned from Casals about playing naturally, which for Mackie meant better use of the self. Mackie found that the Alexander Technique taught her to "let it happen" and saw how that was what Casals inspired in her. The first third of the book recounts her initial training and her work with Casals. The bulk of the text describes the discovery process of making the link between Casals's teachings and the Alexander Technique. Mackie explains that she saw how Casals made her aware of herself when working with an Alexander Technique teacher who improved her through this awareness process. The last portion of the book builds on Mackie's understanding of the links between teaching, Casals wisdom, and the application of these teachings to cello music, especially a lengthy discussion of Bach.

McEvenue, Kelly. *The Actor and the Alexander Technique.* New York: Palgrave MacMillan, 2001.

Kelly McEvenue is an Alexander Technique teacher with the Stratford Festival Theatre in Stratford, Canada. She trained with Frank Ottiwell at the American Center for the Alexander Technique in San Francisco. This text is organized into five parts. The first part is a brief introduction to F. M. Alexander and the Alexander Technique. The four main parts focus on how the principles of the Alexander Technique apply to acting and stage work. In part 1, "The Alexander Technique in the Theatre," McEvenue explains that the Alexander Teacher's role in production of a play is to solve the actors' movement problems as well as explore the physical problems that come from portraying a character. She provides an in-depth discussion of the fundamental concepts of the Alexander Technique, such as recognition of habit, inhibition, and primary control, and also describes basic and relevant anatomical concepts. McEvenue always begins her lessons with a warm-up, and the text's instruction on specific applications also begins in this first part with a description of doing those warm-ups. In part 2, the author describes specific movement applications and exercises. She labels these "partner work and spatial awareness exercises." These are designed to provide a sense of the three-dimensional, voluminous body and its spatial presence on stage. Each of the eight exercises are specific activities with step-by-step explanations. In part 3, the author discusses the Alexander Technique and voice work. While this is a relatively short essay, compared to the other sections, she provides her unique perspective into voice issues for musical theater and opera singers, as well as a whispered "ah" exercise. In the last section, "The Alexander Technique and Acting Challenges," McEvenue discusses how the Alexander Technique can benefit specific acting events and movement requirements such as (1) kissing, (2) nudity, (3) falling and fainting in stage, (4) drunkenness, (5) martial arts, and (6) playing another gender. She includes a valuable lesson on the actor and fitness. Finally, she describes how the actor adapts to playing the space on different types of stages, including (1) the Proscenium-arch stage, (2) the raked stage, (3) the thrust stage, (4) theater in the round, and (5) outdoor theater.

Potter, Nicole, ed. *Movement for Actors.* **New York: Allworth Press, 2002.**
Nicole Potter has assembled over twenty-three articles and essays on physical
movement in acting skills, their effect on the body, and how to improve movement on stage. Techniques and concepts include the Alexander Technique and the
integrated actor, the Feldenkrais Method, the Laban movement, and "breathe before you act," in the section on "body basics." Other discussions include the Meyerhold system of actor training, the Williamson physical technique, the Margolis
Method, and the "Actor as Athlete of the Emotions: The Rasaboxes Exercises."
In the discussion of the Alexander Technique, written by Teresa Lee of the drama
department at Appalachian State University, she concentrates her points on "acting with ease," that is, changing the fixed habits that interfere with daily life
through the use of the primary concepts of the Alexander Technique, including
sensory appreciation, primary control, and conscious direction. Beyond description of the origins of the Alexander Technique and basic definitions, Lee describes a typical lesson for actors.

Priest, Julia. *From Stage-fright to Seat-height: An Annotated Bibliography
on the Alexander Technique and Music, 1907–1992.* **North Grosvenordale,
Conn.: Author, 1992.**
This self-published book consists of selected articles, books, and dissertations
and theses on the Alexander Technique, with a particular focus in music. There
are three primary sections: (1) Articles, including journal articles published as
early as 1907 and as late as 1992, (2) Books published between 1979 and 1991,
and (3) Dissertations and theses published between 1974 and 1993. There are
only five books in the "books" section, but there are fourteen dissertations and
theses and 112 articles. Each entry has a paragraph-length annotation, though
some of these paragraphs are very short. Priest also provides a two-page guide on
how to locate the publications listed and a detailed subject index.

Sherman, Mozelle Clark. *The Great Teachers: Interviews with 20/21st
Century Teachers of Voice and the Alexander Technique.* **N.p.: Sherman,
2002.**
This text reproduces a double-spaced, typed manuscript of the author's recorded
interviews with six noted voice teachers, including Anna Kaskas, Arthur New-
man, Esther Hinds, Peter Trimmer, Elena Nikolaidi, and Jay Wilkey. Each section
features one of the voice teachers and includes a biography of that teacher, an introduction that the author uses to explain the inclusion of that particularly voice
teacher and the relevance of their expertise to the subject, the dialogue recorded
during the conversation, and black-and-white diagrams of physical and vocal exercises. Each of the six teachers discuss instruction in vocal training, including
body use, the Alexander Technique principles, and applications of these principles. The text also includes a "physiological appendix," an illustrated anatomical
manual defining the thorax, axis and atlas, oral cavity and pharynx, mandible, vocal folds and muscles of the larynx, trachea, and nasal cavity.

32

Chapter 2

ARTICLES

Almeida, John, and James Shugart. "The Action in Akron: The 1993 ITG Conference." *ITG Journal*, 18, no. 1 (1993): 4–27.
The authors provide a detailed description of the workshops, programs, and activities of the 1993 International Trumpet Guild Conference held in Akron, Ohio, in 1993. There are four sections in the article: (1) Recitals, (2) Lecture-Demonstrations, (3) Concerts, and (4) Student Competition. There is only one report on an Alexander Technique program in the "Lecture-Demonstrations" section of the article. A one-page description recounts the offering of Barbara Conable on the Alexander Technique. The session began with a performance of the Northwestern University Trumpet Ensemble. Conable then explains her work with musicians and the purpose of the Alexander Technique. She provided more specific discussions on working with trumpet players, noting that about one-tenth of all trumpet players drag the whole pelvis forward in a kind of brace, which causes the jaw to tighten, which then affects embouchure formation. Conable then applied lessons to several students in attendance on the stage.

Babits, Linda, and Hillary Mayers. "The Path to Productive Practicing: An Introduction to the Alexander Technique." *American Music Teacher* 38, no. 2 (November/December 1988): 24–26.
The authors posit the argument that the Alexander Technique can make practicing in music lessons a "more engaging, creative and ultimately productive activity." A brief discussion of F. M. Alexander and his technique segues into how learning to observe oneself in detail during practice can develop the capacity to focus on one thing at a time, no matter how small, to become interested in it and overcome boredom during practice. The authors argue that "this brings about a deep mindfulness and a focus akin to what people sometimes experience in meditation." This kind of focus causes the musician to think and listen differently. Instead of thinking about what has failed in musical output, the student thinks about what is happening with body movement during musical performance, in a "spirit of adventure" that allows the student to isolate and identify problems. The process eventually leads to the capacity to slow down and creates a newfound patience. The authors also describe the history and mission of the North American Society of Teachers of the Alexander Technique (NASTAT).

Barker, Sarah A. "The Alexander Technique: An Acting Approach." *Theatre Topics* 12, no. 1 (March 2002): 35–48.
The author poses a substantial premise that the actor's power to use thought to change physical use and to approach the region of the subconscious is a significant benefit of Alexander Technique instruction. She describes in extensive detail three fundamental self-use objectives of the Alexander Technique applicable to theater and acting, including (1) reduction of excess physical compression and muscularity for physical ease, (2) the unification of body/voice and thought, and

(3) expansion of the field attention. This article begins with substantial background material on the application of Alexander Technique in theater and acting instruction. However, the bulk of the article delves into the properties and benefits of the three self-use objectives. Sarah Barker describes the issue of "physical ease" from an anecdote told by Anne Bogart, which describes the paradox of creating greater ease in movement. This often results in a profound sense of conflict and tension in a character on stage. Barker describes how the Alexander Technique can be combined with a physical exploration of the characters psychology to create a greater psychological depth. She also describes similar applications of the Alexander Technique for dealing with the constraints often experienced by young actors in what could be called "fighting energy" from the difficulty of performing restricted movements. The author also argues that Alexander Technique instruction bolsters "somatic unification" by eliminating excess tension and bringing the whole body into conscious awareness. She notes that the Alexander Technique can help an actor reach a physical state sensitized to emotional and psychological conditions to create a stronger sense of reality. Lastly, Barker states that actors using the technique's "expanding the field of attention" are able to achieve a stronger stage presence by inclusion of the audience and the theater space within their consciousness.

Batson, Glenna. "Conscious Use of the Human Body in Movement: The Peripheral Neuro-anatomic Basis of the Alexander Technique." *Medical Problems of Performing Artists* **11, no. 1 (March 1996): 3–12.**
The author "discusses the peripheral neuro-anatomic basis for the Alexander Technique: the role played by the body's proprioceptors (the peri- and intraarticular neural afferents) in movement organization." Proprioceptive training, which is a form of reeducation used in orthopedic and sports medicine rehabilitation, is compared and contrasted with the Alexander Technique principles in depth. Glenna Batson argues that Alexander must have known of the study of proprioception, though he never mentions it, because of the significant parallels in Alexander's method of self-teaching approach to posture and movement at the exact time scientific theories on proprioception were being developed. For example, Alexander focused on methods of releasing tension patterns in the neck just when neurophysiologists discovered massive numbers of muscle spindles in the cervical musculature. Batson also describes the history of proprioception, which in today's connotation relates just to posture and position, and kinesthesia, which concerns a sense of movement. The scientific work in this field involves the study of various afferent neurons called "mechanoreceptors" in and around the joint capsules, which act as transducers, converting a specific physical stimulus into a neural pulse. Batson explains how Alexander's work has transformed human movement science from the theory that individual receptors act as regulators of proprioception and movement to a theory centered in a systems approach to motor control and motor learning.

————. "Stretching Technique: A Somatic Learning Model. II: Training Purposivity through Sweigard Ideokinesis International." *Impulse: The International Journal of Dance, Science, Medicine, and Education* 2, no. 1 (January 1994): 39–58.

Stretching techniques are an integral part of training in dance science, and
dance instructors have long recognized the benefit of somatic education to
dancers in developing good stretching technique. Dance science is seen as offering safe and effective stretching through teaching the behavioral properties
of muscle and connective tissue, while somatics emphasizes sensory respon-
sivity and motor organization for purposive action in the dancer's work and
training. Purposivity is a necessary component of this training to ensure directional intent. In this work, usage is compared in two models of neuromuscular
reeducation: Alexander Technique and Sweigard Ideokinesis. The author provides a description of the methods for stretching the hamstrings using ideoki-
netic imagery. This is seen as adding anatomical and biomechanical specificity
to the Alexandrian experience.

Ben-Or, Nelly. "The Alexander Technique and Performance." In *Tensions
in the Performance of Music,* ed. Carola Grindea, 84–95. London: Kahn &
Averill, 1985.

Nelly Ben-Or describes the basic principles of the Alexander Technique in depth.
Her primary focus is to show the reader how it is important to learn to alter the
patterns learned in music instruction. Ben-Or argues that it is also important to
distinguish "infusing intensity" not tension into any piano technique.

Beret, Arcaya. "Teaching a Singing Monkey." *NASTAT News* 1 (Summer
1987): 4.

Arcaya Beret describes the implementation of the Alexander Technique activity
known as "the monkey" that teachers can use to help singers improve their physical well-being and vocal abilities. There are basic and easy-to-understand
anatomical explanations, as well as a description of chair work. The "monkey" to
open up breathing is a central part of the article. The author emphasizes the use
of mirrors to practice the technique.

Bosanquet, Caroline R. "The Alexander Principle and Its Importance to
Music Education." *British Journal of Music Education* 4, no. 3 (November
1987): 229–42.

The author provides a useful and practical discussion of the application of the
Alexander Technique for cellists and singers. The article has a primary focus on
methods for improving posture while performing. There is an extensive discussion of tension management as well. One of the more useful components of the
article delves into the improvement of tonal quality through Alexander Technique
instruction and application of its principles. Caroline Bosanquet also promotes
the technique as a benefit for nonmusicians.

Bosch, Amanda, and John Hinch. "The Application of the Alexander Technique to Flute Teaching: Two Case Studies." *British Journal of Music Education* **16, no. 3 (1999): 245–71.**

The authors describe through two case studies how the Alexander Technique was employed to improve the performance of two individual flute players. Each student had different levels of capabilities and progress in their skill and instructional level, and were of different ages. The various tensions exhibited by each student are described in detail and the solution sought. Specific Alexander Technique applications are documented, especially as regarding the improvement of tonal quality. There is a brief description of the Alexander Technique's historical background and an explanation of the authors' qualifications as musicians and Alexander Technique teachers. Case 1 concerns an advanced amateur flutist who exhibited a strained and thin tone when she attempted to play louder. She often complained of fatigue and lower back pain as well. The Alexander Technique exploration discovered that she held her head back too far with arms too far front, with shoulder blades up and tense. Instruction included getting the student to release weight into the sitting bones, relaxing the buttocks, movements to release the tension in the neck. The second student was new to the flute. She held her neck, arms, and flute in an awkward position, pulling and lifting her left shoulder higher than her right. Breathing instruction from Alexander Technique instruction did improve the student's breathing, but other aspects of the technique proved too difficult for this young student.

Buchanan, Heather J. "On the Voice: An Introduction to Body Mapping: Enhancing Musical Performance through Somatic Pedagogy." *Choral Journal* **45, no. 7 (February 2005): 95–101.**

The author focuses on improving musical performance through body mapping, an integral concept of somatic education, of which the Alexander Technique is one such educational method. Body mapping centers on mind-body coordination and the freedom of movement through this relationship. Body mapping is a significant component of Alexander Technique training. Heather Buchanan begins by discussing the need for body mapping, how it can be useful for musicians, and the importance of moving the body in ways to avoid injury. The basic principals of body mapping and training the senses as it relates to being more responsive are a significant component of her article. This work also includes the more physical aspects of body mapping including training the core muscles of the body, balance, and breathing. Buchanan emphasizes that body mapping has been viewed as an effective supplemental tool for teaching music students and describes several simple exercises to improve musicians' public performance skills. There are tables that outline some of the exercises and information on the spine, the senses, and places of balance in the body.

Calder, Lelia. "The Alexander Work." *NATS Bulletin* **42, no. 3 (January/ February 1986): 19–21.**

Lelia Calder argues that the Alexander Technique's primary value is in how it can teach an individual to direct attention to the body as a psychophysical unit and aid them in retraining faulty movement patterns used in basic activities, especially walking, sitting, and standing. She explains that the technique is a hands-on instructional method with verbal instruction that must be done within a classroom, school setting, or teacher's studio. The author notes that the most important tenet, known as "primary control," is coordination of the head, neck, and back and that is essential to the technique's instruction and success. Alexander Technique instruction also emphasizes that students need to learn to inhibit the unconscious repetition of bad habits. This will provide the ability to restore alignment and flexibility. As the individual's reeducation progresses, improvements in breathing ability are realized and then reintegrated with the central nervous system. Calder describes these principles within the context of vocal training.

Conniff, Richard. "For Young Actors, Tisch Is the School of Hard Knocks."
***Smithsonian* 19, no. 6 (September 1988): 55–67.**
The author chronicles a day of acting lessons at the Tisch School of the Arts at New York University. The day is the final day before a three-school acting competition between the Tisch, Yale School of Drama, and the Juilliard School. Richard Conniff warmly describes the very human interaction between teachers and students learning to overcome their shortcomings and build their acting skills. Enunciating correctly is one issue, and slouching on stage is another. For the latter, Ann Matthews is introduced as the Alexander Technique teacher, who notes that the lessons build self-awareness so that actors can rebuild their body for a more natural effect. This discussion on the Alexander Technique is relatively brief, but the story gives a more humanized view of struggling actors in training.

Connington, Bill. "The Alexander Technique: Learn to Use Your Body with Ease." ***Massage Magazine* 63 (September/October 1996): 20–24.**
Bill Connington describes the benefits of the Alexander Technique in conjunction with massage therapy. He begins by telling the story of two massage therapists who incorporate the Alexander Technique in their massage sessions, one who is the massage therapist for the opera singers at the Metropolitan Opera. Connington describes how the Alexander Technique is used by massage therapists in their own use of their body-work sessions, offering advice such as how to bend over the massage table. He also briefly describes the fundamentals of the Alexander Technique, especially the importance of the head, neck, and spine relationship. The author notes that the Alexander Technique is sought after by a wide variety of people, from the performing arts to sports and for general health concerns. He goes into a thorough description of a typical session as well. Connington makes a final plea to the reader to show that it is a useful tool for massage therapists.

Dawson, William J. "Ask the Doctor: Treatment Options for Medical Problems. II." ***Double Reed* 28, no. 2 (2005): 145–47.**
This feature is a regular column in this journal. In this column, William Dawson describes several "physical treatment methods" he indicates are classified as "integrative medicine" within the medical profession and suggests they may be use-

ful therapies for double reed musicians. He divides these therapies into four categories: (1) manual therapy, including physical therapy and massage therapy; (2) topical therapy, or applying substances to the skin, such as aspirinlike compounds; (3) body awareness methods, including the Alexander Technique, Feldenkrais, and yoga; and (4) acupuncture, including reflexology. The discussion of the Alexander Technique is brief, two short paragraphs, but Dawson notes that the Alexander Technique teacher teaches the student to recognize and "unlearn: established adult posture patterns that produce stress and pain."

de Alcantara, Pedro. "In a Spin." *Strad* 114, no. 1360 (August 2003): 832–37.
The author is a widely published, internationally noted cellist and advocate of the Alexander Technique, especially for cellists. He studied the cello for a time with Pablo Casals and has written of the inspirations, including the Alexander Technique, he realized from these experiences. In this article, he builds an analogy of cello performance to that of jugglers in a Chinese circus, where coordinating the spinning of plates on a pole is likened to the coordination needed for the whole body, "learning left hand and bowing techniques, interpreting the musical text, and interacting with colleagues, conductor and audience." In the article, Pedro deAlcantara uses stories of cellists to illustrate the need for the benefits of the Alexander Technique for coordinating the body while playing the cello. The article includes color photographs illustrating some of the instructional methods. He also provides a discussion on the proper way to analyze someone's coordination. There is also a discussion of ideal bodily position when playing the cello.

Dorrit, Frederick. "Music and Movement." *Clarinet and Saxophone* 30, no. 3 (Fall 2005): 35–36.
In this brief article, the author describes the benefits of the Alexander Technique for musical performance, especially for clarinet and saxophone. He describes the different attitudes musicians exhibit toward movement and posture. His discussion describes both the Alexander Technique and hypnotherapy as useful forms of improving posture and body movement for performance enhancement, and compares the two methods and their value to the performer.

Elman, Darcy. "The Alexander Technique." *Share Guide* 5, no. 2 (Winter 1994): 17.
Darcy Elman is a cheerleader for the Alexander Technique in this article promoting its value to dancers. She describes her experiences as a dancer who overcame tension, stress, and pain after taking Alexander Technique lessons. She notes that her introduction to the Alexander Technique occurred while watching dancers who were studying the technique; she noticed they danced with joy and looseness, something she felt she had lost. Elman states that some people describe the Alexander Technique as an approach to correcting posture, but she sees it as much greater than that, able to relieve tension, build energy, and aid people in reaching their potential. She describes its main principles briefly, as well.

Evans, Nigel. "Alexander Technique: An Introduction and Bibliography of Recommended Resources for the Musician." *Brio: Journal of the United Kingdom Branch of the International Association of Music Libraries, Archives and Documentation Centres* 37, no. 1 (Spring/Summer 2000): 9–12. See music library for copy.

Farkas, Alexander. "Coach's Notebook . . . Exploring the Alexander Technique and Opera." *Opera Journal* 28, no. 3 (September 1995): 16–22.
Alexander Farkas takes the reader through an extensive discussion of how the Alexander Technique can improve opera performance. He explains how the Alexander Technique can inform the portrayal of characters, their personality, and emotions in opera by describing how it can improve the performance of the Countess Cavalina Porgi amor scene, the opening scene in Act II of Mozart's Le Nozze di Figaro. Farkas explains how three Alexander Technique tenets are key to this process, including "nondoing," "the means-whereby," and "end-gaining." Farkas notes that the Alexander Technique creates the ability for the operatic performer to obtain a simplicity in performance where the demands of portraying emotional states on stage cause such physical and mental challenges and stress. Farkas also states that the Countess Cavalina scene often suffers a certain amount of excessive emotional and physical heaviness vocally, emotionally, and musically. The remainder of the article, then, attempts to explain how "nondoing" is an energetic process of taking away awareness that tells the performer what is unnecessary. To achieve a portrayal of the suffering of the countess, the singer must perform from a state of physical well-being, with buoyancy and expansiveness. Farkas believes that some of the technique, especially "means-whereby," cannot be truly transmitted in print but requires hands-on instruction.

Fleezanis, Jorja, and Jon Bernie. "A Different Kind of Practice: Musicians and the Alexander Technique." *Strings: The Magazine for Players and Makers of Bowed Instruments* 4 (July/August 1989): 31–34.
Jorja Fleezanis, an Alexander Technique teacher, recounts a conversation between himself and his student, Jon Bernie, a string instrumentalist. The conversation details the step-by-step process Fleezanis uses in his instruction of the technique. The dialogue shows the interaction between teacher and student and demonstrates the challenges of teaching and learning the technique.

Fortin, S., W. Long, and M. Lord. "'Three Voices' Researching How Somatic Education Informs Contemporary Dance Technique Classes." *Research in Dance Education* 3, no. 2 (December 1, 2002): 155–79.
This paper reports the findings of an ethnographic research project on the educational value of the Feldenkrais Method. The authors recognize the Alexander Technique as another somatic education method, in addition to the Feldenkrais, but do not employ it in this study. Their research examined how the Feldenkrais, as a somatic educational method, improves or aids (1) transfer of learning, (2)

movement awareness facilitation, and (3) construction of the dancing bodies. Their findings suggest the need for a shift in dance culture where self-awareness in dance is common practice. They imply that the Alexander Technique, as a somatic educational method, has implications for similar results.

Friedman, Jonathan. "Reflections on the Alexander Technique." *Interlude: Official Journal of the Boston Musicians' Association and the Boston Musicians' Building Association* **(July/August 1991): 7–8.**
Jonathan Friedman provides an excellent and readable introduction to the Alexander Technique and all of its basic principles. He is an enthusiastic promoter of the technique, which is clearly seen in his lively style of explanations. Friedman demonstrates examples of applications with musicians as a means for explaining each principle in relation to musicians' work.

Haigh, Charles. "Gathering of the Clans." *Strad* **107, no. 1272 (April 1996): 394–96.**
Charles Haigh provides a lively and readable account of the "Gathering of Clans" festival held October 1995 in Leeds, an annual gathering of British cello teachers and their students. The article describes the events of the four-day festival and the enthusiasm of the participants for its offerings, especially footage of some of the great cellists, Pablo Casals, Emanuel Feuermann, Andre Navarra, and Mstislav Rostropovich. The festival included master classes with Alexander Baillie and Amanda Truelove as well as individual teachers. The article briefly describes the Alexander Technique lessons given by Vivien Mackie, and describes how to apply it in practice.

Hanson, Rebekah. "Repetitive Injuries in String Musicians." *American Suzuki Journal* **33 (Fall 2004): 79–82.**
Rebekah Hanson notes that research on repetitive strain injuries among musicians has been limited but that awareness of the problem is growing rapidly. She describes the history and progression research on this topic before detailing specific injuries. The bulk of Hanson's article details the symptoms and causes of several different types of repetitive injuries, including (1) repetitive strain injury, (2) playing-related musculoskeletal disorders, (3) tendonitis, (4) tenosynovitis, and (5) carpal tunnel syndrome. Hanson then describes the benefits of the Alexander Technique and Feldenkrais Method for prevention and relief of these repetitive strain disorders.

Harper, Nancy Lee. "The Definitive Solution Is Surgery." *Healing Alternatives for Musicians, in American Music Teacher* **44 (April/May 1995): 8–11.**
The author describes her struggle with carpal tunnel syndrome while working on a degree in piano performance and with the medical profession that saw surgery as the only solution. Seeking to avoid the debilitating consequences of this invasive course, she discovered the benefits of acupuncture and discusses the benefits she received from this therapy. Her experiences led to an exploration of other alternative

therapies. In this article, Harper provides a basic description of several of these methods, including the Alexander Technique, acupressure, Feldenkrais, osteopathy and chiropractic procedures, applied kinesiology, homeopathy, and otho-bionomy. In her coverage of the Alexander Technique, she lists the seven basic movements of the Alexander Technique.

Heirich, Jane R. "The Alexander Technique and Voice Pedagogy." *NATS Journal* 49, no. 5 (May/June 1993): 16–19.
The author provides a brief biography and history of F. M. Alexander and the Alexander Technique, then makes the case that the Alexander Technique is "not about release of tension per se, but about efficiency of muscular use (i.e., appropriate use of the appropriate muscles at the moment for whatever the task)." For Jane Heirich, it is not a relaxation technique but rather is about balanced strength, coordination, and ease of movement. She describes five basic principles, including (1) a human being is a working unity and must be treated as a whole, (2) a great many of our problems are the direct result of how to do what we do, (3) what is familiar feels "right," (4) the working of the human organism is guided by what Alexander called "primary control," and (5) an Alexander lesson is a process of reeducation. She then describes her observations from the teaching studio, such as (1) vocal nodules are frequently the result of systematic behavioral patterns and not just a problem arising from misuse for which the Alexander Technique can uncover systematic interferences, and (2) incomplete closure of vocal folds causing pressed phonation and weakness of the voice can be due to collapsed posture as well as abusive vocal usage and stress, which can be improved by the Alexander Technique to redirect energy and correct posture.

———. "Supporting the Voice." *NASTAT News* 3 (Winter 1988): 1, 4.
Heirich describes and explains a Dart procedure sequence, beginning with creeping through the activity known as "the monkey" and ending with vertical movement. Her purpose in the article was to demonstrate the integration of primary control into the support of the voice. Heirich gives more explanations of the Alexander Technique principles and its value to vocal pedagogy as well.

Heringman, Jacob. "The Alexander Technique and the Lute." *Lute News: The Lute Society Magazine* 73 (April 2005): 7–18.
Jacob Heringman describes the teaching and application of the Alexander Technique as it relates to lute practice and performance. He concentrates on explaining seven central concepts of the Alexander Technique, including primary control, inhibition, direction of use, the function of the organism as a whole, means and ends, the effect of use on functioning, and the unreliability of sensory appreciation. This article is one of a rare few that describes lute performance instruction with the benefits of the Alexander Technique.

Hudson, Barbara. "The Effects of the Alexander Technique on Respiratory System of the Singer/Actor; Part 1: F. M. Alexander and Concepts of His Technique that Affect Respiration in Singers/Actors." *Journal of Singing* **59, no. 1 (September/October 2002): 9–17.**

The author investigates how the Alexander Technique influences respiration, especially for singers and actors, through the three primary instructions of rediscovery of the upright reflex, primary control, and the movement of the spine. After detailing the biography of F. M. Alexander, his theories of respiratory reeducation in two of his works, *Man's Supreme Inheritance* and *Constructive Conscious Control*, are described. She notes that Alexander was known as "the breathing man" and that he was keenly aware of the importance of breathing. Alexander believed that an understanding of true principles of atmospheric pressure and how they work, within the lungs, the equilibrium of the body, the center of gravity, and the line primary movement in each component of the breathing mechanism was necessary. Barbara Hudson describes, in depth, several Alexander Technique concepts that effect respiration, including primary control, development of the upright reflexes and the concept of body mapping. She also details how red muscle fibers, which are ideal for maintaining the appropriate curve of the lower back, important to lengthening the body, can lose their use from people not using them to deal with gravity correctly and that this will lead to slower and deeper respiratory movement. She also discusses the respiratory and expiratory phases examined under Alexander Technique body use. A second article on the implications for training respiration in singers and actors follows in the November/December issue of the journal.

————. "The Effects of the Alexander Technique on Respiratory System of the Singer/Actor; Part 2: Implications for Training Respiration in Singers/Actors Based on the Concepts of the Alexander Technique." *Journal of Singing* **59, no. 2 (November/December 2002): 105–10.**

This article continues the author's work from part 1 published in the previous issue (September/October 2002). Hudson begins by discussing the lack of research on the use of the Alexander Technique in the teaching of singing, noting that its origins from Alexander's acting background tended to steer more research efforts to that discipline. She also believes that research on this topic is sparse because the Alexander Technique demands more sensory awareness than traditional vocal training. However, Hudson found a growing body of work in recent years that examines Alexander Technique training for singers, discussing, especially, the work of Gwyneth Lloyd, a singer, opera director, and Alexander Technique teacher from South Africa. Hudson goes on to describe and discuss several aspects, for singers, of the application of the Alexander Technique that lend themselves to research and further study. Some of these topics include (1) posture versus upright reflexes, (2) field of attention, (3) unlearning previously learned habits, (4) focus on expiration and back movement, and (5) end-gaining.

Iammateo, Enzo. "The Alexander Technique: Improving the Balance." *Performing Arts and Entertainment in Canada* **30, no. 3 (Fall 1996): 37.**
The author describes the benefits of the Alexander Technique to performing artists, appealing to readers in Canada by recounting a conversation with Boaz Freeman, a Toronto Alexander Technique teacher. Freeman notes he first learned of the technique from a violin builder he met while studying in London. Freeman describes the technique as a means for identifying muscle tension while creating a balance between head, neck, and back. A brief history of the Alexander Technique is also described. The author also suggests that the Alexander Technique increases energy through the reduction of muscle tension, which helps in daily activities as well as aids in better breathing.

Isley-Farmer, Christine. "The Private Studio: Legs to Sing On: A Practical Guide for Singers and Voice Teachers." *Journal of Singing: The Official Journal of the National Association of Teachers of Singing* **61, no. 3 (January/February 2005): 293–99.**
Christine Isley-Farmer provides a very useful discussion of the relationship of the feet, legs, and lower torso to the overall support mechanism for vocal training and singing performance. She uses the Alexander Technique to explore its application and value to improving lower body problems. There is an excellent inclusion of practical applications based on the Alexander Technique as well as other bodywork modalities. Isley-Farmer utilizes a number of anatomical and visual aids and describes several movement concepts to improve the learning experience for students. She also promotes the Aston-Patterning technique to help singers with improving their physical health and ability at standing on stage. She explains how this technique shows that, by not locking the body, three-dimensional movement on stage can be facilitated. The author describes and promotes other concepts developed by Judith Aston, especially her belief that human movement occurs in asymmetrical and three-dimensional spirals. Exercises based on Aston's work are also included.

Kosminsky, Jane. "The Alexander Technique." *Ballet Review* **23 (Summer 1995): 92–94.**
Jane Kosminsky uses this article to promote investigation of two well-known Alexander Technique texts to dancers. She notes that it is hard to describe experience as a way of helping dancers overcome their reluctance to read the difficult subjects of the books but argues that these deal with the subject exceptionally well. The two texts are *The Alexander Technique: The Essential Writings of F. Matthias Alexander*, selected and introduced by Edward Maisel, and *The Alexander Technique* by Judith Leibowitz. Kosminsky extols Maisel's introduction as a very illuminating treatise on what is important about the Alexander writings, all of which are included in his book. She notes that all the most famous passages are included in the text, such as the cases of the stutterer and the golfer who couldn't keep his eye on the ball. Kosminsky tells the reader to substitute "dancer" for "golfer" to get a better picture of

why dancers struggle with alignment. In her discussion of Leibowitz's book, the author explains that Leibowitz and her coauthor, Bill Connington, tell the "how" of the technique and that the Leibowitz Procedures, a simple series of movements such as lifting the arms and bending the knees, are also explained step-by-step.

Lautenschalger, N., et al. "Physical and Mental Practices of Music Students as They Relate to the Occurrence of Music-Related Injuries." *Work* **6, no. 1 (January 1996): 11–24.**
This research was predicated on previous research conducted at the New England Conservatory in Boston. The authors sought to record the general physical and mental habits of music students and to determine if there were any associations between these habits and the appearances of music-related injuries. Three hundred music students at Boston University were given a questionnaire, with forty-five responding, giving a return rate of 15 percent. General findings recorded include (1) 68 percent of female and 53 percent of the males reported a music-related injury, (2) most reported they played their instruments even when experiencing some pain, (3) 61 percent reported visiting with more than one type of rehabilitation specialist, which included Alexander or Feldenkrais teachers, (4) 52 percent reported reacting well to stress, and (5) 44 percent reported having an average level of self-consciousness. The authors concluded that the data on lifestyles of musicians was valuable to rehabilitation specialists in treating musicians but that musicians needed more information about available rehabilitation treatments.

Lewis, Pamela Payne. "Teaching the Technique for Academic Credit." *NASTAT News* **12 (Summer 1991): 10–11.**
Pamela Lewis advocates for developing creditworthy courses on the Alexander Technique in college and university music schools and programs. She describes what she believes are important components to a college-level course on the technique for engaging students' verbal, visual, and kinesthetic learning styles and requirements. The article includes quotes from her students who have taken her courses on the technique.

Mackie, Vivien. "The Alexander Technique and the Professional Musician." *Interlude: Official Journal of the Boston Musicians' Association and the Boston Musicians' Building Association* **(July/August 1990): 20–22.**
This article was originally published in the *European String Teachers' Association Journal* and reproduced, with some revisions, in this journal. Vivien Mackie describes the basic principles of the Alexander Technique within the context of music instruction.

Madden, Catherine. "The Language of Teaching Coordination: Suzuki Training Meets the Alexander Technique." *Theatre Topics* **12, no. 1 (March 2002): 49–61.**
The author explains her experience integrating Alexander Technique instruction with Suzuki training for theater students. Suzuki training in this context is not to

Chapter 2

be confused with Suzuki violin training but rather is a Japanese form of teaching stage actors to "walk" in a stylized way—hips, knees, and ankles in bent parallel position, stomping at each step. Designed by Tadashi Suzuki, this form of movement training is designed to strengthen the connection between voice and movement and the power of the whole body to speak, even when the voice is silent. It increases physical and vocal strength. Catherine Madden found that language choices in teaching Suzuki can be improved through three strategies. First, anatomically accurate description of movement is more effective than nonanatomical images. Second, performers' coordination deteriorates when they confuse muscle contraction with thought processes. Third, students today have an "electronic language," and this appears to interfere with psychophysical processes. The author describes the history and background of the Suzuki training method and the Alexander Technique, and melds these two discussions so complementary aspects are compared and explained in context. Madden then describes in detail the precise anatomical language necessary to make Suzuki training, aided by Alexander Technique, effective, and argues for "anatomical accuracy" in instruction. She defines in a clear way terms, including (1) upper body/lower body, (2) leg movement, and (3) the "abs" and the arms, and describes how tradition and Suzuki training contributes to "mismappings." She also discusses the issues caused by Suzuki instruction on thought processes and how it is important to separate these from muscular action. For example, in Suzuki, the concept of "fighting spirit" can produce excess muscle work and the Suzuki concept "concentrate" can often result in face and eye tightening. Madden makes the case that the Alexander Technique can be used to help adjust muscle contraction by applying lessons from psychophysical perspectives and describes strategies for four prime Suzuki thought processes. Lastly, she describes strategies for dealing with the "electronic language" of today's students.

Malocsay, Rosemary. "Know Thyself . . . and Thy Student." *American String Teacher* **38 (Winter1988): 77.**
In this brief article, Rosemary Malocsay, a music teacher, discusses the process of teaching and building quality in one's instruction. She advocates the integration of the Alexander Technique in music instruction as important to prevent injuries and a remedy for stress and pain. She quotes Alexander Murray on "tuning the player."

Mayers, Hillary, and Linda Babits. "A Balanced Approach: The Alexander Technique." *Music Educator's Journal* **74, no. 3 (November 1987): 51–54.**
The authors argue that the Alexander Technique is a "reduction of habitual movement patterns so the body is used efficiently with the least amount of wear and tear" as a preventive technique for dealing with physical problems in performance such as carpal tunnel syndrome, tendonitis, and chronic muscle spasm. They describe the fundamentals as a threefold process of (1) the development of an awareness of the body's physical state, (2) the conscious decision not to re-

spond to a situation in a habitual manner, or (3) teaching how to organize the body through a series of clear mental instructions regarding balance of its parts, also known as "direction." Each part of this process is briefly described, but the authors caution that the process can only be learned through hands-on instruction. A very clear before and after photo demonstrates the posture in vocal performance. The authors describe the application of the technique and list the advantages and benefits.

McGovern, Mary. "Spinal Comfort." *Strad* **110, no. 1311 (July 1999): 724–25.**
Mary McGovern discusses ways of finding a suitable position for holding a violin or viola for practice and performance by learning the Alexander Technique concept of "primary control." She discusses several common problems in holding the violin or viola and then gives advice on applying the Alexander Technique to learn better posture. There is a step-by-step exercise provided to help with placing the instrument in position. Her advice includes adjusting the shoulder and chin rests to allow the head and shoulder to support the instrument without the shoulder coming up toward the ear and placing the head in contact with the chin rest without losing the full length of the neck and back.

Mnatzaganian, Sarah. "Behind the Scenes: Magic Hands." *Strad* **113, no. 1350 (October 1, 2002): 1160.**
This article is a regularly featured column and presents the views of Graham Griffiths, a violinist with the Royal Philharmonic Orchestra and an Alexander Technique instructor for the Royal Academy of Music in London. Griffiths describes his experiences as an Alexander Technique teacher with orchestra instrumentalists. He discusses how a "more efficient and natural use of the body in standing, sitting and walking" is related to playing and expounds upon his students reactions to his instructions, mostly positive. He relates an anecdote where he eased the tension in the back of a famous conductor (unnamed in the article) who later rejected the instructions because his style of conducting was based on tension.

Myers, Martha, with interviews by Margaret Pierpont. "Body Therapies and the Modern Dancer." *Dance Magazine* **57 (August 1983): BT9–BT11.**
In this special pull-out section of *Dance Magazine*, the authors describe and discuss several methods of body therapy and interview several professionals in this field as these therapies relate to dance. The prime therapies with a separate article include the Alexander Technique, Feldenkrais, and the Bartenieff Fundamentals. Interviews with dance professionals on other ideas and therapies include Remy Charlip, Norma Leistko, Martha Myers, and Todd Sweigard (Ideokinesis). The article on the Alexander Technique does not include an interview with an Alexander Technique teacher. However, the author describes the origins of the technique and explains some fundamental concepts, especially primary control, inhibition issues, and automatic body behavior as a "set." In "Using the technique," she tells of her own experience in Alexander Technique lessons. She explains the importance of

the role of teacher in helping students discover how, on their particular body, articulation of the head, neck, back, or ribs may contribute to faulty initiation of a body movement. The author argues that learning the Alexander Technique is as much about how each student learns, a state of mind, as what is learned. The author promotes dancers "taking the risk" to allow the movement to happen to explain how it works.

Naylor, John. "The Alexander Technique: From Pupil to Teacher." *Music Teacher* **68 (April 1989): 19–20.**
John Naylor describes the benefits of the Alexander Technique to piano instruction. He argues that the Alexander Technique aids pianists with hand-crossing, awkward reaches, and figurations. He discusses methods for piano teachers for integrating the technique into their instruction.

Nesmith, David. "How Body Mapping and the Alexander Technique Will Improve Your Playing." *Bass World* **26, no. 2 (October 2002–January 2003): 24–25. Also in** *International Musician* **99 (June 2001): 11.**
David Nesmith argues that the body is our instrument and that if the body is "pinched or tense, our sound will be pinched or tense." He goes on to describe somatics as the study of the body in motion and notes there are two tools to discuss that aid in the understanding of somatics, body mapping, and the Alexander Technique. He provides an explanation of both in the remainder of the article.

Nix, John. "Developing Critical Listening and Observational Skills in Young Voice Teachers." *Journal of Singing* **59, no. 1 (September/October 2002): 27–30.**
John Nix begins with a humorous, personal anecdote to demonstrate that vocal teachers often do not know the source of the problems of their students. Too often a general approach that asks them to do more of what they don't understand is the tact. Nix asks the question, "What needs to be changed or added to the current training curriculum in order for young voice teachers to learn how to diagnose the causes of vocal problems?" He then proposes several activities and instructional concepts that address this question. One of these ideas is instruction on body awareness activity. Nix suggests this should be the Alexander Technique, Feldenkrais, or yoga. He found that whole body awareness methods, including the Alexander Technique, are effective in assisting voice teachers in understanding and interpreting sympathetic body responses. Other activities he describes include guided listening/videotape viewing sessions, independent listening study, and using a voice assessment instrument, among others.

Norris, Richard. "Overuse Injuries: How String Players Can Recognize, Prevent, and Treat Them." *Strings: The Magazine for Players and Makers of Bowed Instruments* **4 (November/December 1989): 45–47.**
Richard Norris describes the problems of repetitive injuries string instrumentalists experience from a medical professional's point of view. His article is not di-

rectly about the Alexander Technique; however, he enthusiastically promotes it as an effective treatment. This article describes the causes of injuries, including instrument ergonomics and various anatomical anomalies, and discusses body mechanics and various body-work techniques. Norris believes that a conservative approach to treatment is best.

Ohrenstein, Dora. "Physical Tension, Awareness Techniques, and Singing." *Journal of Singing* **56, no. 1 (September/October 1999): 23–25.**
The author poses the question "Why do many singers make strange faces when they perform?" She notes her own self-discovery process while attempting to answer this question and found that physical tensions must be addressed in addition to the act of singing to make real, deep-lasting changes in one's physical habits. She describes how the Alexander Technique and Feldenkrais are techniques to help the singer let go of old habits because it is difficult to do this on one's own. Dora Ohrenstein describes her experiences in depth, with the Feldenkrais. She found audiotapes that were designed to help sufferers of temporomandibular joint (TMJ) syndrome based on the Feldenkrais that were quite effective. She explains some of these exercises as well. The author discusses how voice teachers do not always realize that great success in relieving tension and building conscious awareness can occur from these techniques when not in conjunction with voice instruction. She promotes these views as represented in Kristin Linklater's book *Freeing the Natural Voice*. Ohrenstein concludes by promoting the idea that voice needs to draw on the Alexander Technique and Feldenkrais, as well as eastern philosophies and contemporary psychology.

Perron, Wendy. "Body Work Approaches Guide." *Dance Magazine* **74, no. 11 (November 2000): 74.**
Wendy Perron notes that the one positive outcome of an injury to a dancer is that it leads to a holistic view of body health. Several alternative and complementary therapies are then listed with a brief annotation. These include the Alexander Technique, Feldenkrais, integrated movement exercise, Klein Technique, Pilates, Skinner Releasing Technique, the Trager Approach, and five more. Perron suggests that the Alexander Technique teaches dancers about how excessive tension is used, causing too much stress in the body, and explains that the technique uses hands-on guidance so that the dancer can learn to relieve pain.

Perron, Wendy, and Karen Hildebrand. "Be Gentle to Your Body." *Dance Magazine* **78, no. 3 (March 2004): 60–62.**
The authors provide a review and explanation of several video recordings and compact disks on dancing and physical fitness. These include *Pilates Mini-Ball Workout with Leslee Bender* from Balanced Body, *Movement Nature Meant with Ruthy Alon, the Feldenkrais Method* from Feldenkrais Resources, *Soundpath* CD, envisioned and produced by Naaz Hosseini (a soundtrack recommended for dance practice), and *The Alexander Technique: Changing Your Life by Changing*

Your Posture, a Lesson with Jane Kosminsky from Wellspring Media. In the review of Kosminsky's video, the authors found the instruction given to actor William Hurt by Kosminsky to be not immediately applicable to dancers but found that it sparks creative application to dance instruction of the technique.

Pooley, Eric. "Diane Verona Gets Physical." *New York* **18 (October 28, 1985): 30.**
This article spotlights Diane Verona, a Juilliard-trained actor of stage and screen. Verona believes that her training taught her that acting is athletic in nature, requiring lots of movement and that creating a character takes bold use of body, voice, and mind. Verona found that the Alexander Technique was able to lengthen her torso, which broadened her abilities and gained her wider roles than she would have without the technique. Most of the article describes her career successes and has less to do with the Alexander Technique than her life story.

Richmond, Phyllis. "The Alexander Technique and Dance Training." *Impulse: The International Journal of Dance, Science, Medicine, and Education* **2, no. 1 (January 1994): 24–38.**
Phyllis Richmond explains how the Alexander Technique is especially applicable to dancers and dance instruction because of the dependence on the high-level functioning of the physical and mental coordination of the body in order to perform well. She argues that dancers can correct inappropriate habits through neuromuscular reorganization through Alexander Technique and facilitate the ability to coordinate, focus, and clarify in dance performance. She gives specific advice on use of the principles of the Alexander Technique within a dance context.

———. "Body and Soul." *Teaching Theatre* **8, no. 1 (Fall 1996): 1–2, 12–14.**
Richmond, an acting teacher for a Stanislavski-based professional actor training program at Southern Methodist University, argues that the Alexander Technique and the Stanislavski method, working in concert, significantly contribute to modern acting training. She found that actors use their consciousness to monitor the process that brings characters to life on stage. Performers use different stimuli, both internal and external, to make the character seem natural, as a real person, not an actor on stage. She explains that actor training involves learning psychological techniques as well as physical techniques. However, as Richmond explains, this process causes the actor to feel stress by pressure to perform and then to need the stress to perform. Additionally, stress causes a response that sometimes includes unwelcome consequences such as muscular tension. Richmond makes a cogent argument for the Alexander Technique in eliminating self-centered tension. She notes that the actor finds the process of character portrayal easier, both physically and mentally. A sidebar explains the development of the Alexander Technique and its fundamentals principles. Richmond relates her experiences coaching a cast of the production of *One Flew over the Cuckoo's Nest*

where the characters must reveal their individual psychological disturbances through idiosyncratic patterns of misuse and distortion. She explains these difficult physical portrayals and how the Alexander Technique aided the actors in their portrayal and benefited their health.

Rosenthal, Eleanor. "The Alexander Technique: What It Is and How It Works." *American Music Teacher* **39, no. 2 (October/November 1989): 24–27, 57 (reprint of an article in** *Medical Problems of Performing Artists* **2, no. 2 (June 1987).**
The author describes the history of the Alexander Technique and states that F. M. Alexander's "objective was to teach people a skill that would help them improve the way they executed all of the activities of their daily lives" not just musical performance. While she acknowledges the concept that the Alexander Technique can improve one's behavior and ability in many different daily activities can be doubted by the casual observer, she argues, "The Alexander Teacher is not expected to be an expert in his student's fields. Instead, he has a different expertise: he knows how people's habits interfere with their functioning, and he knows how to help them overcome those habits." Eleanor Rosenthal notes that the Alexander Technique has applications for improving posture and body mechanics, voice, and breathing; reducing or preventing muscle spasms and problems such a chronic lower back, neck, and shoulder pain; and improving mental awareness and emotional well-being. She argues that the magic of the technique is that conscious and unconscious level, and she provides a detailed description of this learning process of the technique. Rosenthal also describes how she applied the technique to music and how the technique improved their conditioning. One student was a violinist whose left shoulder constantly locked causing pain. The second violinist suffered from disabling shoulder spasms. A third student was a pianist who experienced significant pain in her left elbow.

Sanders, Joseph. "Freedom to Breathe." *Strad* **113, no. 1346 (June 2002): 630–32.**
Joseph Sanders begins this discussion of how the Alexander Technique improves breathing capacity and ability by arguing that breathing naturally is a must for any actor or performer that suffers from stage fright. He then goes on to develop the case for learning to breathe naturally, through the Alexander Technique, for string instrument performers, noting that it may not be seen as an obvious advantage for these musicians. However, he notes that the habits of most string instrumentalists are to suck in their breath or some other way of forcing breathing when they begin. He goes on to show the process of string performance has significant use of breath capacity and idiosyncrasies that effect performance. He then provides a seven-step exercise, formulated through the principles of the Alexander Technique, to build the ability to breathe naturally as a string instrumentalist. He also describes the benefits of breathing for preventing stage fright.

Shryer, Donna. "Practical Musician: Music and Musicians—Zing Went the Strings of (Ahh) My Neck: Simple Routines to Keep String Players Ready for Action." *Strings* 20, no. 4 (November 2005): 22, 24–26.
The author provides a detailed description of Jonathan Cole's warm-up and stretching routine for violinists. This routine includes front arm-raises, side arm-raises, shoulder shrugs, chest expansion, bicep curls, shoulder circles, forearm rotation, vertical wrist bends, horizontal wrist bends, and finger spreads. Donna Shryer cautions that these warm-up and cool-down stretches are not meant to improve or alleviate repetitive motion injuries or muscle damage. However, she notes they can relieve tension, tightness, or muscle stress, and there is some evidence that, in the long run, it may prevent injury overall. Shryer relates the work of Cole with that of the Alexander Technique as well.

Sjoquist, Matthew. "Using Massage and Bodywork to Forge a New Mentality for Business." *Massage and Bodywork* 13, no. 1 (Spring 1998): 122–24.
Matthew Sjoquist reviews the success of Higher Octave Music, a recording label, as a business that provides its employees with Alexander Technique lessons and massage on a weekly basis. The owners met at an Alexander Technique session and formed their business on the principle of reducing employee stress to build productivity. The author interviews the owners and several employees on their belief of the viability of Alexander Technique lessons and massage as a business practice.

Stein, Charles Jay. "The Alexander Technique: Its Basic Principles Applied to the Teaching of String Instruments." *American String Teacher* 49, no. 3 (August 1999): 72–77.
The author describes how beneficial Alexander Technique training can be to students of string instruments. Repeated movements in playing strings cause problems with pain and discomfort. Alexander Technique instruction can show students where they are tensing and how to improve their posture to reduce such problems. The article is organized by the primary terminology an Alexander Technique instructor would use, including balancing, directing, grounding, inhibition, opposition, and ends and means. In "balances," Charles Stein explains, for example, "the Alexander Technique teacher sees the body as always being in constant flow and movement and sees good posture as an upward flow and downward flow." He also discusses how violinists try to hold a particular position with their shoulder girdle but the Alexander Technique can show how the skeleton can support the musculature rather than the musculature locking to support the skeleton. Other discussions include directing and how it can show the student the way to release the neck and lengthen the spine just before the body goes into movement while playing a stringed instrument and how important the legs are as well as the arms in playing, especially in connecting to the floor, chair, or both.

Stevens, John. "Keeping Students Dancing: Dance Injury Prevention in Practice." In *Dancing in the Millennium: Proceedings of the Society of Dance History Scholars,* **comp. Juliette Willis and Janice D. LaPointe-Crump, 400–403. Washington, D.C.: Dancing in the Millennium, 2000.**
This publication reproduces the proceedings of "Dancing in the Millennium," an international conference held in Washington, D.C., in July of 2000 and sponsored by a number of dance organizations including the Dance Critics Association, the National Dance Association, and the Congress on Research in Dance, among others. In his paper on the Alexander Technique, John Stevens describes how the dance program at De Montfort University implements the Alexander Technique as an integral component of dance instruction and the benefits of the technique in preventing injuries among students.

Taber, Judith. "Head to the Neck." *Dance Spirit* **7, no. 1 (January 2003): 30–31.**
The author notes that dancers often find themselves stuck in movement patterns that are uncomfortable. She describes how movement control affects this and how it develops from natural and automatic reflexes at birth that change as people get older and shape them to fit their own patterns. She describes the primary postural and muscle organizing reflexes as the head-neck reflexes. A description of a startle reflex and its effect is also provided. Judith Taber then argues that the Alexander Technique builds movement consciousness. She provides a brief history of the Alexander Technique and then a description of a typical Alexander Technique lesson. Three fundamental principles are also briefly defined: (1) expanded consciousness, (2) inhibition, and (3) primary control. Finally, she instructs the reader on how to explore these principles on their own with some easy-to-follow exercises, such as placing the hand behind the neck and head and observing what they do as you stand up. Each exercise is accompanied by a color photoset demonstrating the exercise.

Trobe, Judith. "The Alexander Technique for Prevention and Treatment with Musicians." In *The Seventh Annual Symposium on Medical Problems of Musicians and Dancers,* **26–29. Snowmass, Colo.: Cleveland Clinic Foundation and Aspen Music Festival, August 3–6, 1989.**
Judith Trobe begins her discussion with a biography of F. M. Alexander. She briefly describes the technique's relation and application to music instruction and performance. The bulk of this article recounts her demonstration of Alexander Technique instruction with a student.

Valentine, Elisabeth R. "Alexander Technique." In *Musical Excellence: Strategies and Techniques to Enhance Performance,* **ed. Aaron Williamon. Oxford: Oxford University Press, 2004.**
Elisabeth Valentine describes and discusses the range of published research on the Alexander Technique, especially that which applies to students in the performing arts and professional musicians. This work explains the technique and its

background before discussing the research that supports it and its benefit to performing artists, especially musicians. Research into specific applications of the technique is included.

———. **"The Alexander Technique for Musicians: Research to Date." In** *Psychology and Performing Arts*, **ed. G. D. Wilson, 239–47. Lisse, The Netherlands: Swets & Zeitlinger, 1991.**
The author begins with a biography of F. M. Alexander and a description of the Alexander Technique's basic principles. She then reviews a number of research studies that examined the efficacy of the technique. She notes that most of the research has concentrated on physiological measurements. She also argues that there has been little research on the behavioral and experiential manifestations of the Alexander Technique and its effectiveness in these areas. Valentine also found that many studies employing the technique have lacked adequate controls, such as random allocation of subjects between treatment and control groups.

———, **et al. "The Effect of Lessons in the Alexander Technique on Music Performance in High and Low Stress Situations."** *Psychology of Music* **23, no. 2 (1995): 129–41.**
This article describes a scientific study of the application of the Alexander Technique in musical performance lessons. Twenty-five students with various instruments, including voice, cello, piano, organ, flute, oboe, clarinet, and trombone, were divided into an experimental and control group on a random basis. Experimental measurements were applied and recorded on four separate occasions, two at low stress points (in class prior to treatment and in class after treatment) and two at high stress points (audition and recital) for students in both groups. The experimental group received fifteen lessons in the Alexander Technique, while the control, though aware of the design and treatment, did not receive any technique instruction. The subjects completed the Eysneck Personality Inventory and the Performance Anxiety Inventory. They also rated their interest in having Alexander Technique lessons. At each of the stress points, all subjects were measured for height and peak flow (peak expiratory flow, a measure of the pressure exerted in forced expiration) because of claims that the Alexander Technique increases the realization of potential height and improves breath control. Subjects' heart rates were also gauged as a measure of arousal under stress. Subjects also self-reported their mood, using the Full Nowlis Mood Adjective checklist. The study found that the main hypothesis, that the Alexander Technique would increase height or peak flow or modulate the increase in mean heart rate under stress, was not proven and no effects were found to be statistically significant. However, the experimental group did show improvement from preclass to postclass relative to control on overall technical quality.

———. **"The Fear of Performance." In** *Musical Performance: A Guide to Understanding*, **ed. John Rink, 168–82. Cambridge: Cambridge University Press, 2002.**
Valentine notes the seriousness of performance anxiety (or stage fright) as a phenomenon for many musicians. She explains that the symptoms may be physiologi-

cal (e.g., rapid heartbeat), behavioral (e.g., trembling), or mental (e.g., negative thoughts and feelings). Many practitioners and teachers believe that a moderate level of anxiety enhances performance, but too much anxiety can be very damaging. Valentine discusses the three factors that contribute to performance anxiety, including personality, task difficulty and mastery, and the situation, such as audience factors, setting amenities, and so on. She then goes on to discuss and describe several methods and therapies for overcoming performance anxiety, ranging from those that rely heavily on physical methods to those that rely mostly on mental control and ability, and including the efficacy of deep breathing, progressive relaxation, systematic desensitization, biofeedback, beta-blockers, imagery, Alexander Technique, and positive thinking as in cognitive behavior therapy, stress inoculation, self-instruction, attention focusing, or appropriate timing of anxiety. Valentine also discusses how performers should evaluate each of the possible approaches for their own use.

Wallace, Helen. "Performance-related Injuries . . . Dark Continent?" *Strad* 102 (May 1991): 396–404.

Helen Wallace describes the state of responses within the medical profession to injuries related to musical performance, and the acceptance or attitudes toward various alternative medicines and therapies. The discussion is framed with an understanding of the Alexander Technique presupposed, but there is a sidebar on the technique that describes the current view of British musicians and music students about the Alexander Technique. Wallace found that, in Britain, there is a growing acceptance of the importance of medical preventive techniques for musicians, including partnerships with doctors and music institutions. She reports on the London College of Music's interdisciplinary clinic that incorporates Alexander Technique instruction.

Washington, Lynn. "The Alexander Technique for String Teachers: William Conable, Ohio State University." *American String Teacher* 41 (Spring 1991): 31.

Lynn Washington recounts an Alexander Technique workshop conducted by William Conable at the AST Congress. Using a group demonstration, Conable showed the effects of primary control on arm freedom and breathing. Washington provides a useful and readable explanation of Conable's work.

Weeks, Janet. "Alexander Technique: Get in Gear." *Dance Magazine* 78, no. 5 (May 2004): 31.

Janet Weeks describes the value of the Alexander Technique by first observing how noted dancers like Mikhail Baryshnikov seemed to dance with such ease. She goes on to describe that dancers must deal with the abuse of their body created by the demands of their work and how Robert Britton, Alexander Technique teacher, relates the trials of dancers to the need for learning to improve their body use through Alexander sessions. Weeks provides a brief discussion of how the technique is taught and a description of some of the basic principles. She also includes a testimonial from Mary Cochran, professor of dance, on the benefits she derived from the technique.

Wilson, Glenn D. "Performance Anxiety." In *The Social Psychology of Music*, ed. David J. Hargreaves and Adrian C. North, 229–45. Oxford: Oxford University Press, 1997.
Glenn Wilson provides a substantial discussion of performance anxiety in musical performers. He notes that it affects between 25 and 50 percent of all musicians. He argues that it is most prevalent amongst individuals with highly neurotic traits, including introverts and those prone to social phobia. Performance anxiety is most often experienced when the performer is in exposed and evaluative situations, such as solo performances and auditions. Wilson found that high levels of mentally induced anxiety, combined with complex task demands, can be quite serious and cause severe problems emotionally as well as in the performance itself. He argues that the most successful approaches combine relaxation training with anxiety inoculation and cognitive restructuring, and goes on to describe the Alexander Technique and hypnotherapy as being the most effective of these types of therapies and instruction. He also describes beta-blockers as a possible therapeutic remedy, especially as a stopgap.

Wilson, Glenn D., and Roland, David. "Performance Anxiety." In *The Science and Psychology of Music Performance: Creative Strategies for Teaching and Learning*, ed. Richard Parncutt and Gary McPherson, 47–61. Oxford: Oxford University Press, 2002.
In this essay, Wilson teams up with David Roland to describe and discuss an updated version of his work reported in the *Social Psychology of Music* in 1997. In addition to the in-depth discussion of the causes and effects of performance anxiety, Wilson and Roland describe preliminary research with hypnotherapy and the Alexander Technique and how this research points to the possible benefits of these therapies on reducing performance anxiety.

Zipperer, Daniel. "A Survey of the Alexander Technique as a Supplement to Voice Production." *Journal of Research in Singing and Applied Vocal Pedagogy* 14, no. 2 (1991): 1–40.
Daniel Zipperer conducted a survey of forty-two professors of voice who had been recognized as influential and highly experienced in vocal pedagogy for his master's thesis at Southern Illinois University. The survey examined the professors' views and use of the Alexander Technique. Almost three-quarters of those surveyed reported that the Alexander Technique had mostly positive effects on singing. However, Zipperer found that the level of understanding of the technique varied greatly among all respondents.

DISSERTATIONS

Boardman, Susan D. "Voice Training for the Musical Theatre Singer (Broadway)." DMA diss., University of Cincinnati, 1987, 149 pages.
In this doctoral study, the author argues that there is a need to develop a standard pedagogy of musical theater singing. She begins by examining the lack of such

pedagogy in the literature and history of musical theater instruction and then describes the demands and requirements for singers in musical theater, especially the vocal and physiological needs. In her final chapter, she proscribes a specific vocal pedagogy applicable to singers in musical theater training. While many of the components of this pedagogy are relevant for direct theater and vocal training, the course of study includes instruction with the Alexander Technique. Other components include (1) musical training, (2) classical vocal techniques interwoven with speech and movement, (3) belting, and (4) diction.

Chabora, Pamela Dawn. "A Descriptive Study of the Application of Research in Neuropsychology to Self-use Training for Actors." PhD diss., Michigan State University, 1994, 267 pages.
This doctoral dissertation examined and analyzed publications and expert opinion on the developments in the field of neuropsychology on their effects of self-use training for actors. The author did a comprehensive analysis of a significant number of relevant publications on neuropsychology and actor training, then interviewed acting professors from three very well-known acting schools, the Tisch School of the Arts, the Julliard School, and the Asolo Center Conservatory of Professional Actor training at Florida State University on the link between neuropsychology and self-use training for actors. Much of this study was informed by the work of Dr. Roger Sperry, a researcher in hemispheric lateralization and specialization and the self-use methods of the Alexander Technique, Feldenkrais, and Sweigard's Ideokinesis. This study concludes that there is a cyclical pattern of how neuropsychological research can inform self-use training for actors.

Dennis, Ronald John. "Musical Performance and Respiratory Function in Wind Instrumentalists: Effects of the Alexander Technique of Musculoskeletal Education." EdD diss., Columbia University Teachers College, 1987, 81 pages.
This doctoral study sought to discover the effect of the Alexander Technique on respiratory functions of young adult wind instrumentalists. Thirteen volunteer subjects were assigned to experimental and control groups, with seven in the experimental group. Data was gathered in pretest and posttest events using two methods: (1) videotapes of the subjects' musical performance and (2) respiratory function measurement with a standard spirometry and maximal static mouth pressures. Twenty Alexander Technique lessons were given to the experimental group subjects. There were four operationally defined dependent variables for musical performance, including posture and movement during nonplaying, posture and movement during playing, breath control, and overall performance. There were several dependent variables for respiratory function, including forced vital capacity, forced expiratory volume, peak expiratory flow, and three other variables. The videotapes were analyzed by six experts with the use of analysis of variance (ANOVA). Respiratory data was analyzed using a t-test. The study found that the control group performed better than the experimental group in maximal voluntary ventilation, and no other significant differences were discovered.

DeVries, Katie Sue. "Movement for Actors and Dancers: The Implications of Modern Dance for Actor Training." MA thesis, American University, 1999, 66 pages.
In this master's thesis, the author promotes the concept that movement techniques and dance aid in training for acting. Four movement-based techniques are described, including the Alexander Technique, Rudolf Laban's Effort-Shape Theory, Etienne Decroux's Corporeal Mime, and Constantin Stanislavski's Method of Physical Action, in terms of their relevance to acting and dance instruction and performance. The author then poses the theory that dance training, in conjunction with these four movement techniques, enables actors to learn their craft more beneficially. Several exercises are also included.

Dimon, Theodore, Jr. "Performing Arts, Pedagogy, and the Work of F. M. Alexander." EdD diss., Harvard University, 1987, 210 pages.
Written by one of the more noted authors on the Alexander Technique today, this doctoral study examines the educational theory of F. M. Alexander, especially as it applies to how we learn to do different skills. Dimon's purpose was to create a method of assessing the relevance of the Alexander Technique to how skills are taught today. The intent of the discussion is twofold: (1) to give Alexander Technique teachers a theoretical perspective to using the technique as a teaching tool and (2) to explore the technique's approach to teaching performing skills. Theodore Dimon's dissertation has three distinct parts: (1) an explanation of the origins of the Alexander Technique and its fundamental principles, (2) how the technique applies to teaching and learning, specifically, and (3) a repertoire of concrete examples that demonstrate the theory of this technique in practice.

Doyle, Gerard. "The Task of the Violinist: Skill, Stress, and the Alexander Technique." Lancaster University (UK), 1984.

Englehart, Robert James. "The Electromyographic Study of Preparatory Set in Singing as Influenced by the Alexander Technique." PhD diss., Ohio State University, 1989, 211 pages.
This doctoral dissertation examined how the Alexander Technique can influence the preparatory set in singing and tone quality. Rhythmic timing and the effects of other forms of training were also examined for how they were influenced by the Alexander Technique. A pretest, posttest control group design was utilized with twenty-three novice singers. Each was measured in the pretest and posttest for surface electromyography (EMG) from three muscles in the neck. Two experimental groups and one control group were formed, with one experimental receiving Alexander Technique lessons and the other experimental group receiving relaxation training. Ten days of treatment, consisting of one-hour sessions of the Alexander Technique or relaxation training were administered, and a posttest of surface EMG scores was given immediately afterward. An ANOVA of the data found that there was no significant difference in tonal quality, but the subjects re-

ceiving Alexander Technique lessons showed significant changes in preparatory set stability and greater consistency in response.

Fedele, Andrea Lynn. "The Alexander Technique: A Basis for Oboe Technique and Performance." A.Mus.D. diss., University of Illinois, Champaign-Urbana, 2003, 280 pages.
This doctoral dissertation conducted survey research to examine how the Alexander Technique can aid in improving oboe instruction and performance and help prevent painful misuse of the body in oboe practice and performance. A survey of seventeen experienced oboists on how they play and teach oboe is included. The objectives of the survey were to measure aspects of posture, use of the hands and arms, embouchure and the jaw, breathing, articulation, and practicing. The survey also gathered data on the types and amount of pain experienced by the performers. The results found that 71 percent experienced pain during performance, especially in the hands and arms, and that the self-reported cause was misuse. In addition to use and misuse issues, the survey recorded the oboists familiarity and experience with the Alexander Technique and found that almost all had at least some exposure to the technique.

Fitzgerald, Lynn E. "Breath: Principles Derived from Eastern and Western Literature and Suggestions for Its Use in Modern Dance." EdD diss., Temple University, 1984, 153 pages.
This doctoral study examined the influences of five Eastern and Western somatic educational techniques on breathing and formulated advice and instruction for breathing during dance performance. The five educational techniques included (1) the Alexander Technique, (2) hatha yoga, (3) tai chi, (4) karate, and (5) bioenergetics. Three breath relationships were studied, breath energy, breath-body, and breath-movement. A number of breathing principles were gleaned from the study of the techniques. The author found, for example, that breathing can be controlled, and because of this principle, it can influence energy, body, and movement. She found that breath patterns can be generated for unifying one's energy, body, and movement statement, among other principle findings. She then provides specific advice to dancers on breath control and abilities during dance performance.

Fowler, Sarah B. "Unspeakable Practices: Meaning and Kinesis in Dance (Alexander Technique, Merleau-Ponty)." PhD diss., Temple University, 1987, 212 pages.
In this PhD dissertation, the author sets out to examine theory of dance performance as movement as people perceive it in the performance. The two theories that are commonly held, kinesthetic response and kinesthetic empathy, are described and discussed. The author then poses the theory that, while kinesthetic response as a theory of how we view dance performance is accurate, we need to revise the view that uses kinesthetic empathy, and that this revision is more fully informed and improved

by an understanding of the Alexander Technique and the theories of Maurice Merleau-Ponty, who argued strongly for the role movement plays in dance and movement performances. The author aims to educate dancers, choreographers, and critics that dance needs to be understood on a kinesthetic basis.

Fritz, Mary Ann. "A Piano Pedagogy of Creative Motion." DMA diss., Southwestern Baptist Theological Seminary, 1998, 145 pages.
In this doctoral study, Mary Ann Fritz describes the benefits of the concept "creative motion," which was developed in the 1920s by Martha Stockton Russell to address relaxation and freedom in musical performance. Russell's work emphasizes attention to the naturally occurring energy in the body and aligning it with the motion of the music. Fritz places this study of creative motion in the context of piano pedagogy. While the study does not utilize the Alexander Technique at all, Fritz devotes part of the first chapter to a comparison of creative motion to other similar movements and techniques, especially the Alexander Technique and the work of Emile Jaques-Dalcroze, as well as Abby Whiteside.

Holm, Carolyn Postma. "Correctives to Breathing Hindrances in Flute Performance, with Emphasis on the Alexander Technique." DMA diss., Southern Baptist Theological Seminary, 1997, 176 pages.
The author of this doctoral study conducted a survey of flutists and their breathing ability. The survey "Hindrances to Breathing of Flute Players" was distributed to a number of flutists at the beginner, intermediate, and mature levels of playing. The survey examined the ability of the instrumentalists to conserve air effectively and efficiently with the understanding that the majority of a flutist's air is lost across the tone hole. A chapter on the physiology of breathing is included as part of the discussion. The application of the Alexander Technique to flute performance is described in detail, along with exercises in its application for this purpose. A chapter on the origins of the Alexander Technique is also included.

Janis, Christine Anne. "Opera Workshop for the Undergraduate: More than Aria Coaching." DMA diss., Ohio State University, 1994, 128 pages.
The author of this doctoral study theorized that opera workshop programs only provide aria coaching and training on performing opera scenes. She conducted a small-scale survey in Ohio of professional singers and found that 70 percent reported only receiving aria coaching and opera performance lessons. Four interviews of opera production–related professionals were also conducted and concluded with the same results. An educational model for opera instruction was then developed that incorporated acting, score study, characterization, body awareness, audition strategies, career management, stag combat, stage makeup, and the Alexander Technique, as well as aria coaching and performance. The educational model is described in depth.

Kaplan, Iris. "The Experience of Pianists Who Have Studied the Alexander Technique: Six Case Studies." PhD diss., New York University, 1994.
This PhD dissertation was completed at New York University under the direction of Professor John Gilbert. Iris Kaplan's stated purpose was to document the experience

of six pianists who have had varying experiences with the Alexander Technique in order to examine the possible benefits to improving the health of pianists. Kaplan argues that little study on the specific application of the Alexander Technique to piano playing exists because of the private nature of the Alexander Technique and the stigma of admitting to having problems. Kaplan asked four research questions: (1) What events or experiences led pianists to the Alexander Technique? (2) How did pianists who received instruction on the Alexander Technique describe their lessons? (3) What did pianists report as to how they incorporated the technique into their playing? and (4) What was the reported impact of the Alexander Technique on piano playing and performing? Kaplan identified six pianists studying or taking lessons with Alexander Technique teachers in the New York City area, with the author's former Alexander Technique teacher and the director of the American Center for the Alexander Technique as gatekeepers to guide in these selections. Using an intensive interview over two to three sessions, the author asked questions she developed from her Alexander Technique experiences, a review of related literature, the initial research questions, and comments made by the participants. Using the sequence funnel approach explained in qualitative research methodology texts, she began with general questions and moved to more focused or specific queries as the interview progressed. Follow-up was conducted to clarify details. Kaplan concluded that the Alexander Technique is useful for dealing with problems of pain, discomfort, tension, and stage fright, and it also provides a model for use in preventing injuries.

Knaub, Mary Beth, and Jill Hartwig. "Body Mapping: An Instructional Strategy for Teaching the Alexander Technique to Music Students." EdD diss., University of Pittsburgh, 1999, 206 pages.
This doctoral study set out to measure the similarities and differences in perception between male and female students in an instrumental music program on the application of the Alexander Technique and body mapping instruction. An equal number of male and female students in five instrumental groups, including (1) clarinet/oboe/bassoon, (2) upper strings, (3) lower strings, (4) pianists, and (5) singers, were asked to keep journals and prepare reports of their instruction on the Alexander Technique and body mapping taught by William Conable, the developer of the body mapping concept. The author then analyzed the journals and reports using the computer program NUD*DIST (Non-numerical Unstructured Data Indexing, Searching, and Theory-building) to organize the data from these journals. The author then analyzed the data and found that there were more similarities than differences between men and women students but that they processed the information in different ways. There is a thorough description of the Alexander Technique, body mapping, and the origins of the technique as well.

Lloyd, Gwyneth. "The Application of the Alexander Technique to the Teaching and Performing of Singing: A Case Study Approach." M.Mus. thesis, Universiteit Stellenbosch (South Africa), 1987, 155 pages.
This master's thesis is a case study approach to examining the effectiveness of the Alexander Technique in singing instruction. A pilot study of one case was the initial

data-gathering point. Five case studies were then recorded. Each singer in the six case studies was assessed for vocal and physical aspects and concerns. Thirty lessons of the Alexander Technique were applied, and then each case study participant provided detailed explanations of their experiences with the interferences that affected the production of vocal sound and the application of muscle reeducation toward reflex-facilitated postural poses. The author provides a brief review of the literature on singing and the Alexander Technique as well.

Lorenz, Steven Robert. "Performance Anxiety within the Secondary Choral Classroom: Effects of the Alexander Technique on Tension in Performance." M.Mus. thesis, Michigan State University, 2002, 91 pages.
In this master's thesis, the author conducted an experimental study on the application of the Alexander Technique in reducing performance anxiety in choral performance. Two groups of high school students in choral ensembles were formed, an experimental and control group each. The experimental group received thirteen lessons of sensory awareness and body alignment exercises based on the Alexander Technique, and the control group received no body-work lessons of any kind. The study found that the efficacy of the technique as an approach to reduce performance anxiety was inclusive but that the same subjects showed positive changes in posture, state of relaxation, breath control, and vocal technique.

McCullogh, Carol Porter. "The Alexander Technique and the Pedagogy of Paul Rolland." DMA diss., Arizona State University, 1996, 107 pages.
Carol McCullogh's dissertation examines the confluence of the teachings of F. M. Alexander and the noted violin scholar Paul Rolland. She begins by noting the influences and connection between the Alexander Technique and string instrument pedagogy. She describes the good use and misuse of the head/neck/back relationship (as defined by Alexander) and includes a number of photographs of violin and viola players to illustrate the primary Alexander Technique principles. McCullogh also describes teaching approaches influenced by the technique. A biography of Paul Rolland is also included, noting that Rolland was a proponent of the Alexander Technique. An annotated bibliography featuring studies pertaining specifically to the performing arts is also provided.

Oliver, Suzanne Kathryn. "Toward Mind/Body Unity: Seeking the Deeper Promise of Dance Education." PhD diss., University of Illinois, Champaign-Urbana, 1994, 172 pages.
The cultural context of the approach to dance instruction and performance is examined in the doctoral dissertation. The author analyzed what she determined to be "polar opposites that characterize Western epistemology" in how people view dance as a cultural value and learning how to dance. Most of this discussion has been informed by the author's study of the Alexander Technique and she sought to redefine her approaches to dance and dance instruction from the principles and benefits of the technique to dancers. There is an extensive discussion of dance theories and also the origins and principles of the Alexander Technique.

Pearson, Eleanor (Lee) May. "What Every Flute Teacher Needs to Know about the Body: A Handbook of Applying the Principles of Body Mapping to Flute Pedagogy." DMA diss., Ohio State University, 2000, 108 pages.
This doctoral dissertation is designed as an anatomical reference handbook, fully illustrated and designed for teachers in musical and other fields. The purpose of the book is to provide a means for learning body mapping as it relates to flute pedagogy for numerous aspects of that instructional purpose. The book includes topics on sitting, standing, hand and arm use, and breathing. Several exercises are included and fully explained that aid students in learning to play the flute with proper body use. There is a significant discussion of body mapping in general.

Rogers, Sandra Margaret. "Survey of Piano Instructors: Awareness and Intervention of Predisposing Factors to Piano-related Injuries." EdD diss., Columbia University Teachers College, 1999, 176 pages.
This doctoral study sought to determine the awareness of predisposing factors of piano-related injuries that piano instructors understood and were able to identify. A survey was mailed to one thousand instructors in independent schools, colleges and universities, and community music schools. The survey asked for the instructors' knowledge of specific types of injuries, possible causes, and the applicability of several body-work methods, such as the Alexander Technique, Feldenkrais, and yoga. The survey realized a return rate of 21 percent, and found that 40 percent of the instructors were highly aware of these predisposing factors of piano-related injuries. These factors included tension, technique, posture, practice habits, stress, repertoire, genetic predisposition, memory, and computer use. It also found that 55 percent of the teachers reported that their students experienced a piano-related injury. Follow-up interviews were also conducted. The author describes strategies for dealing with these injuries.

Sella, David. "An Application of Selected Body Structure and Postures of the Human Body to the Fundamentals of Cello Technique." PhD diss., New York University, 1981, 132 pages.
This doctoral study examined the body-work aspects of cello playing and how to improve them. The author interviewed several professionals with expertise in either cello performance or body-work techniques, including a professional cellist, a teacher of cello, an Alexander Technique teacher, a physician, and a physiotherapist, to evaluate a number of sitting postures for their effect on muscle tension and body movement. Problems identified included chair height, neck tilts, back collapse, leg and feet postures, and other conditions. The study suggested ways for improving body movement and posture during cello practice and performance.

Sullivan, Claudia Norene. "Movement Training for the Actor: A Twentieth Century Comparison and Analysis." PhD diss., University of Colorado, Boulder, 1987, 213 pages.
This doctoral dissertation provides a historical review and analysis of the trends and theories of movement training in acting instruction. The author begins by

examining the history of body use and training from the primitive times, through ancient Greece, and on to the rhetorical acting of the seventeenth century. A significant portion of the work describes the principles and ideas developed by Constantin Stanislavski, Vsevolod Meyerhold, and Jerzy Grotowski. Stanislavski's "Method of Physical Action" is seen as the most useful. The dissertation then describes and discusses three nontheater body-work and movement training methods, including (1) the Alexander Technique, (2) the Feldenkrais Method, and (3) Rudolf Laban's Effort-Shape Theory. These discussions are formulated within their applications to acting training. The author concludes with the present-day needs for movement training.

Tillman, Rochele Ann. "Voice and Body Incorporated into Actor Training." MA thesis, University of Nevada, Las Vegas, 1999, 87 pages.

This master's thesis examines both vocal and physical training aspects for actors and combines the techniques in a single-class instructional model. The vocal training styles of three well-known instructors, Edith Skinner, Cicely Barry, and Kristin Linklater, are compared and applied in the first part of the instructional design. Several body-work methods are then examined and analyzed for inclusive principles, including the Alexander Technique, Laban Neutral Mask work, tai chi, and modern dance. The final product integrates important aspects of these instructional methods into an acting class.

Wabich, John Christopher. "The Practical Application of the F. M. Alexander Technique to the Performing Percussionist." MM thesis, California State University, Long Beach, 1992, 44 pages.

This master's thesis is designed to inform percussionists about the benefits of the Alexander Technique to their performance and health. The author uses percussion performance experiences to illustrate the principles of the technique. He begins with an explanation of the origins of the Alexander Technique and its main principles. Then, the application of the technique to specific percussion movements is illustrated.

Weiss, Maria Ursala. "The Alexander Technique and the Art of Teaching Voice." DMA diss., Boston University, 2005, 350 pages.

In this doctoral dissertation, the author compares the Alexander Technique in the application of voice instruction to other body-work techniques. She begins with a thorough review of literature on the Alexander Technique and vocal pedagogy, citing such experts as Pietro Francesco Tosi, Manuel Garcia, Kristin Linklater, and Olga Averino, and she includes a review of vocal teachers who are Alexander teachers as well, such as Jane Heirich and Beret Arcaya. Additionally, she discusses the principles of the Alexander Technique as a comparison to other mind-body-work methods, especially Feldenkrais. In a different section of the thesis, she describes the aspects of the technique as it relates to posture, breathing, practicing, and performing, and within the context of other mind-body techniques, especially tai chi and the breathing work of Carl Stough. There is a detailed discussion of the anatomical relationships to posture and breathing.

Zipperer, Daniel M. "A Survey of the Alexander Technique as a Supplement to Voice Instruction." M.Mus. thesis, Southern Illinois University, 1989.
Zipperer conducted a survey of forty-two professors of voice who had been recognized as influential and highly experienced in vocal pedagogy for his master's thesis at Southern Illinois University. The survey examined the professors' views and use of the Alexander Technique. Almost three-quarters of those surveyed reported that the Alexander Technique had mostly positive effects on singing. However, Zipperer found that the level of understanding of the technique varied greatly among all respondents.

3

Resources for Sports, Fitness, and Recreation

The resources in this chapter address specific issues in sports, fitness, and recreation, particularly swimming, running, and physical exercise. The Alexander Technique has been an effective technique in sports and fitness activities in significant ways. It aids in improving breathing, stretching, and lengthening the torso, skills that enhance sports and fitness ability. The Alexander Technique also helps individuals reeducate themselves about proper posture and movement habits that are crucial for many sports' activities, and relieves pain, tension, and stress in the back, neck, and spine. Some of the resources included are from specific sports publications with a substantial coverage of that sport. Other resources, especially some of the magazine articles, are known as general and popular magazines for sports enthusiasts and athletes, and the articles in these magazines tend to be brief and designed for the purpose of promoting the awareness of the Alexander Technique to a general audience that may be interested in sports in general. In the "books" section of this chapter, one entry does not include an annotation. This book was not available through lending libraries, especially those with access through the Online Computer Library Center (OCLC) online database. Most of these publications are from foreign sources and may be available in European or other world libraries. They have been included here to identify them as possible sources useful in learning more about the Alexander Technique.

BOOKS

Balk, Makolm, and Andrew Shields. *The Art of Running with the Alexander Technique*. London: Ashgrove Publishing, 2000.
This work describes how the Alexander Technique can be applied to running to improve for sport and competition, as well as to keep the body healthy. The authors,

Makolm Balk and Andrew Shields, are long-distance runners who discovered the benefits of the Alexander Technique in other venues, Balk from cello lessons and Shields from swimming. Both authors tell their story of getting into the sport of running and how the Alexander Technique came to improve their health and abilities. They provide a brief history of the Alexander Technique, in the context of imagining Alexander as a runner rather than a public speaker. They also explain the fundamentals of the technique, especially primary control, faulty sensory awareness, recognition of the force of habit, inhibition, and direction. They use stories and analogies from the running world to aid in these discussions. Throughout the book, other runners tell their story as a way of illustrating concepts. The authors give their view of fitness and why running benefits fitness in two chapters, including a discussion of holistic fitness. The core of the text describes (1) how to run well, a treatise on good and bad running characteristics in general and (2) how the Alexander Technique can be applied to improve running skills. For example, they discuss "running tall," with eyes forward, putting one's leg in front of the other, with stability in the torso (called head-neck-back relationship in the Alexander Technique). Breathing, freeing the arms and legs, and double-spiral patterns are other discussions. The text also provides "drills for Alexandrian runners," including (1) high knees while avoiding neck tightening or spine shortening and maintaining your full length, (2) high knees at the bottom of a hill, (3) bum kicks (run slowly and allow heels to kick your bum), and (4) step-overs.

Bentley, Joni. *Riding Success without Stress*. London: J. A. Allen, 1999.
Joni Bentley describes the benefits of applying the Alexander Technique to riding and equestrian arts. She argues, "The Alexander Technique brings more brilliance, ease of movement and grace to riding and it is only a matter of time before it shines through the horse world. After all, how can horses be calm, straight and forward with crooked and tense riders?" She also explains that advanced movements demanded by a rider, which in trick riding can be brutal on the horse if performed with a rider with poor posture, are vastly improved by the Alexander Technique. Throughout the first half of the book, Bentley explains the fundamentals of the technique, always using riding examples and analogies to illustrate the concept. Each of the chapters is fully illustrated with color graphics or photographs. For example, to describe "primary control," a discussion with diagrams of balancing on a saddle is used to advance this concept. In part 2 of the book, specific exercises and lessons on horseback riding are described using Alexander Technique principles and techniques to describe how to improve that aspect of riding. These topics include: (1) the dressage seat, (2) listening legs, (3) building context, (4) rising trot, (5) sitting trot, and (6) canter, along with discussions of how relaxation aids in riding.

Gorman, David. *On Fitness: Extracts from a Conversation with David Gorman*. London: Learning Methods, 2000.

Rickover, Robert M. *Fitness without Stress: A Guide to the Alexander Technique*. Portland, Oreg.: Metamorphous Press, 1988.

Robert Rickover relates two incidents of men who were dedicated to fitness but died due to poor health decisions, specifically the wrong kind of exercise, to illustrate that there is a difference between fitness and health. He analyzes the history of problematic approaches over the last forty years, then argues that a completely different approach to fitness is needed, from one of quantity of exertion to one of quality of our movements, that is, balance and coordination, which he describes as the challenge to the fitness myth. Rickover then describes how the Alexander Technique is essential to proper fitness. He explains that misuse of the body causes abnormal pressures on joints and the vertebrae, distorts body shape, and obstructs the operation of vital organs. In exercise, muscles can be overly contracted, locking whole areas of the body into fixed positions, forcing the body to expend more energy in harmful ways and causing chronic fatigue and other weakenings of the body's defense system. Rickover describes how the Alexander Technique prevents and improves these conditions for better health and exercise. He includes descriptions of a typical Alexander Technique lesson, how to locate a certified teacher, and recent developments and applications of the Alexander Technique in other fields.

Shaw, Steven. *Master the Art of Swimming.* London: Collins & Brown, 2006.
Steven Shaw's work explains and illustrates his method of swimming and building swimming skills. His course on swimming was developed by applying the principles of the Alexander Technique, especially the central idea that the relationship between head, neck, and back is responsible for the body's overall coordination. Shaw begins with his own story of his trials and tribulations in competitive swimming. Shaw was an avid swimmer in his youth but became burnt out due to lack of successful competition. After discovering the Alexander Technique while studying political theory and the connection between thought and action, he rekindled his interest in swimming. His first chapter explains the method of swimming based on the Alexander Technique. For example, he explains the basics of swimming in Alexander Technique terms, such as "primary control," which Shaw explains as paying attention to form and allowing the head to lead the rest of the body as the best way to resolve specific stroke faults. In his chapter "Fundamentals: Core Practices," he begins with a significant discussion of swimming basics fully informed by the Alexander Technique, especially breathing, but also buoyancy, balance and stability, resistance, and efficient swimming. The final three chapters are robust descriptions of specific swimming strokes and movement, including the breaststroke, the crawl, and the butterfly stroke. The book is fully illustrated with a large number of color photograph sets.

Shaw, Steven, and Armand D'Angour. *The Art of Swimming: A New Direction Using the Alexander Technique.* London: Ashgrove Publishing, 1996.
This work is designed to improve the abilities of swimmers. Each chapter describes and explains swimming concepts and skills. However, the authors firmly believe that the Alexander Technique has direct beneficial relevance to building

swimming ability and interweave the application of the Alexander Technique into each discussion. There is a beginning chapter that describes the origins and fundamental principles of the Alexander Technique, but the authors add how to apply these fundamentals to learning how to swim. In one of the most important chapters, the authors describe the psychological barriers to swimming. In this chapter, they discuss letting go of the fear that is so often brought to children by adults. Children have natural poise in the water, but traditional training instills these fears. The authors found that the Alexander Technique encourages a sense of continual exploration and self-discovery. Breathing naturally is a significant aspect of the Alexander Technique, and proper breathing is crucial to successful swimming skills. The authors not only describe basic breathing applications from the Alexander Technique but also explain specific adaptations for specific swimming strokes. Also described in one chapter, leading with the head and how the Alexander Technique addresses this body movement for swimmers is demonstrated with photographs and graphics. How these can be applied to specific swimming strokes is also included. The authors end with a treatise on proper fitness and warn of the damaging effects of swimming using bad habits.

Tottle, Sally A. *Body Sense: Revolutionizing Your Riding with the Alexander Technique*. North Pomfret, Vt.: Trafalgar Square Publishing, 1998.
Sally Tottle describes and explains the purpose and components of her "Body Sense" course, an instructional plan to teach horseback riders how to apply the Alexander Technique to improve their balance and body control while riding. Using case histories and black-and-white photographs and graphics, Tottle gives specific advice on how to integrate the Alexander Technique in riding lessons. Tottle is an Alexander Technique teacher whose clients come from many disciplines, but her interest came from an injury that affected her horsemanship. A first lesson is described as a work locating the atlanto-occipital joint and showing the student the habits of misuse that affect this, breathing excess tension and other joints. A chapter on the fundamentals, including the concepts of primary control, use of the self, inhibition, directions, and gaining are discussed using riding examples. Specific instruction on use and misuse of body and position as it relates to riding is also described, including locating the joints in taking rein contact, lower-arm awareness, and hip joint, lower leg and foot, and ankle joint awareness. An extensive discussion of the seat bones describes Alexander Technique applications for sitting in a saddle for balance and poise. The whispered "ah" is described to aid in breathing. There is also a lengthy discussion of the Alexander Technique and riding styles, including racing, show jumping, and cross-country jumping. The "Body Sense" course Tottle developed emphasizes training your horse as you train yourself. Tottle promotes understanding the kinesthetic sense of riding, a monitoring of tension through receptors in the joints, muscles, and tendons. This kinesthetic sense relies heavily on sensory awareness the Alexander Technique can teach. This process also requires the rider to communicate this sense with the horse in which the back plays a crucial role.

ARTICLES

Eller, Daryn. "Workouts that Fight Stress." *American Health* **13, no. 4 (May 1994): 72–77.**
The author describes her evolution from exercise classes and videos designed to build muscle or lose weight to her exploration of mind-body fitness techniques. She notes that these techniques claim to promote harmony, increase pleasure, and reduce mental stress, which drew her to her investigation since the workout exercises she had experienced seemed to create stress and were not relaxing. She describes some of her experiences, especially with Pilates, NIA Technique (neuromuscular integrative action), and Laban/Bartenieff. She discusses the benefits and drawbacks of mind-body workouts. In one sidebar, she details six exercises for relaxation, including a knee drop, arm circle, and abdominal curl. In another sidebar, she provides a guide to seven mind-body techniques including the Alexander Technique, NIA, Feldenkrais, Pilates, Laban/Bartenieff, Yokibics, and Warriorbics. The annotation for each is brief, stating its core purpose, a very brief history, and where to get more information.

Evans, Rory. "Posture Perfect: There's a Reason Why Everyone's Talking about Pilates and Other Ways to Straighten Up." *Women's Sports and Fitness* **20, no. 5 (June 1998): 122–25.**
The author describes, in commonsense language, how good posture is important to health and fitness. He discusses different views, from chiropractors to physicians, why people exhibit poor posture, relating much of this in a discussion of everyday lifestyles and activities. The discussion is a relatively brief, one-page narrative with a brief mention of the Alexander Technique. The narrative is then followed by two pages of color photograph sets demonstrating at least one aspect of the Alexander Technique, Feldenkrais, and Pilates methods. For the Alexander Technique, sitting on a chair and the "monkey" are illustrated.

Ives, Jeffrey C., and Jacon Sosnoff. "Beyond the Mind-Body Exercise Hype." *Physician and Sportsmedicine* **28, no. 3 (March 2000): 67–81.**
The authors begin by noting that many of the mind-body techniques (which they call "exercise methods") and their claims are not supported by clinical evidence. Because they are alternative therapies, legal and professional ramifications of this lack of clinical evidence need to be understood. After defining what mind-body technique (exercise methods) is, which they explain as the mind-body connection of thoughts, emotions, attitudes, and behaviors affecting physiologic function, they describe the scientific evidence that exists for five mind-body therapies, including (1) the Alexander Technique, (2) yoga, (3) tai chi, (4) Feldenkrais, and (5) Pilates. For the Alexander Technique, the authors state that few controlled trial studies exist, but evidence does seem to suggest that it promotes low stress levels and elevates mood states. The remainder of the article describes issues for practice by medical professionals who consider these therapies for their patients,

including issues of contraindication, liability risk, and philosophical conflicts, among other aspects.

Keresey, Maggie. "Stay Limber Longer: Here's How to Keep the Spring in Your Step for Years to Come." *New Choices* **38, no. 4 (May 1998): 32–36.**
The author makes a commonsense argument that individuals need to choose a consistent exercise and fitness program that fits their own criteria and lifestyle. She then goes on to describe six programs worth considering for health and fitness, including the Alexander Technique, ballet exercise, yoga, Pilates, tai chi, and the Feldenkrais. Each of the six program descriptions is formatted with six questions, answered briefly, including what it is, how it works, what you wear, benefits, drawbacks, and cost. Alexander Technique benefits listed include improving coordination and flexibility, and drawbacks listed include that practitioners are concentrated in more populous urban areas and may be hard to locate.

Milios, Rita. "Old Habits Die Hard." *American Fitness* **19, no. 5 (September/October 2001): 30–32.**
Rita Milios appeals to fitness trainers in this article on the Alexander Technique. After a brief discussion of the history of the Alexander Technique, she notes that the technique has two main principles: (1) inhibiting old, patterned, habitual reactions and (2) redirecting the body into alternative responses. The author describes what happens in a lesson, quoting Nancy Crego, an Alexander Technique teacher. She explains that a typical lesson set lasts for thirty individual sessions, and students are taught first to learn to stop the misuse of their body. Crego offers some commonsense suggestions for fitness trainers in the article. She explains that trainers need to pay attention to a client's head, neck, and back to make sure they move in a single line while exercising. Use of a towel or mat under the client's head during floor exercises is also recommended to help with alignment.

Rhodes, Maura. "Wind Down Workout." *Health* **21 (February 1989): 50–51.**
This short article includes one page of text and one page with a photoset illustrating the workout. The author is a "movement consultant" and certified Alexander Technique teacher. She promotes the technique as a mind-body method for becoming aware of and changing habits that can cause tension and pain. The workout is described in eleven steps. These are very specific movements beginning with "lie on back, feet flat, fingertips resting on hip joints" to "reach with right arm to lead right side of body back onto bed."

Rhodes, Maura, and Jack Gescheidt. "Complementary Exercise." *Women's Sports and Fitness* **17, no. 1 (February 1995): 45–50.**
The authors recount the story of Vicki Poth, manager of Barney's Gymnasium and Spa in New York, who suffered severe hip and knee tension while training for the New York City marathon. Poth used Pilates lessons to build balance strength in both of her quads and hamstrings, relieving pressure on her joints. The author describes five complementary techniques athletes can use to restore equilibrium in their body, build a mind-body awareness of themselves, and prevent

strain due to tension and misuse. For swimmers, she discusses how the Alexander Technique can benefit the athlete in swimming skills and breathing. The other techniques described are (1) yoga for runners, (2) Pilates for skiers, (3) tai chi for hikers, and (4) Feldenkrais for cyclists. Each entry answers three questions: (1) what it is, (2) what it is like, and (3) how it can improve the specific sport described. For the Alexander Technique for swimmers, the authors explain that the technique stresses the importance of unfolding and lengthening the torso, which swimmers need to do well. The Alexander Technique can also improve breathing, also very beneficial to swimmers. A photoset accompanies the entry on the Alexander Technique demonstrating the lengthening of the torso in swimming.

Shaw, Steven. "Alexander Technique and Swimming." *Positive Health,* **no. 31 (August 1998): 56–60.**
Shaw reports that a study by the American Swimming Coaches Association (ASCA) found that less than 5 percent of swimmers are able to swim far enough and fast enough to improve their aerobic capacity. He promotes the concept of swimming with a good technique can improve breathing and health, and reduce stress; he also promotes his "Shaw Method of Swimming" as the technique for achieving this. After an anecdote about his own childhood swimming experiences, he describes how he learned about and benefited from the Alexander Technique. He provides a useful discussion of how to apply the Alexander Technique to swimming training, describing more than four specific activities, including (1) recognition of habit, (2) demonstration, (3) guidance, and (4) breaking down the stroke. He devotes a significant portion of the final discussion on the importance of breathing and how the technique aids in this process.

DISSERTATION

Krim, Don. "Multiple Perspectives on the Experience and Effectiveness of the Alexander Technique in Relation to Athletic Performance Enhancement: A Qualitative Study." MS thesis, California State University, Fullerton, 1993, 191 pages.
This master's degree study was designed as a qualitative examination of the value of the Alexander Technique to athletes and sports performance. An in-depth interview was conducted of five athletes who have studied the Alexander Technique. The interviews were structured as open-ended phone interviews. The data collected through the interviews were then analyzed with an inductive content analysis method. This analysis resulted in the data being grouped into two broad categories: (1) experiential, including (a) awareness, (b) wholeness, (c) control, (d) mastery, and (e) confidence; and (2) effect, including (a) stress management, (b) injury prevention and recovery, and (c) learning. The study concluded that the Alexander Technique benefits athletic performance in several ways. The author also compares the results reported through this analysis with peak experiences reported in the literature.

4

Resources for Health and Medicine

The Alexander Technique has not always been received within professional medical circles as readily as within the performing arts. The technique is often considered an "alternate" or "complementary" therapy. Beginning with the promotion of the technique by Raymond Dart, a South African anatomist and anthropologist, the medical profession slowly began examining the effects and benefits of the Alexander Technique for a variety of medical conditions. Medical and health applications include aid for women in birth and pregnancy, research into relief of Parkinson's disease, easing of pain and stress, especially back pain, and improvement of mental health, among other health uses. The resources listed below present works from a diverse set of publications. Some are serious medical and research journals, while others are popular literature mass-marketed to a growing health-conscious public. Some of the entries come from alternative and complementary health magazines as well. A search of *Dissertations Abstracts International* did not reveal any dissertations or theses in a medical field that utilized the Alexander Technique in the study.

BOOKS

Bassman, Lynette, ed. *The Whole Mind: The Definitive Guide to Complementary Treatments for Mind, Mood, and Emotion.* Novato, Calif.: New World Library, 1998.
Lynette Bassman argues that mainstream psychotherapy ignores the potential benefits of a large array of alternative therapies and fails to fully inform mental health consumers of the choice and possible benefits of these therapies. The bulk of her text describes over thirty-four therapies and activities and how their applications could potentially be beneficial for various mental health concerns. Some

of these activities and alternative therapies include the Alexander Technique, Rolfing, the Trager Approach, aromatherapy, and yoga. A wide range of other discussions include topics from homeopathy to Edgar Cayce on mental health, just to mention a few. The article on the Alexander Technique is written by Joan Arnold, who describes the basic technique and answers the major questions including what the research shows, what to expect in an Alexander Technique session, and how to find a practitioner.

Berjeron-Oliver, Sherry, and Bruce Oliver. *Working without Pain: Eliminate Repetitive Strain Injuries with the Alexander Technique.* **Chico, Calif.: Pacific Institute for the Alexander Technique, 1997.**
The authors have designed a text to combat repetitive strain injuries (RSI), such as carpal tunnel syndrome and others, through the integration of the Alexander Technique in work and everyday life. They make a strong case that ergonomics is not enough to overcome these RSI syndromes but that the fundamentals of the technique in learning proper habits of standing, sitting, and other activities maximizes the efficiency of ergonomics and reduces or eliminates RSI at a greater level. The first three chapters describe the problems of RSI, including the risk factors affecting the body, psychosocial stress impact, and definitions of most of the RSI syndromes, including tension neck syndrome, thoracic outlet syndrome, epicondylitis, carpal tunnel syndrome, herniated and deteriorated disks, and sciatica and low back pain. All of these discussions fully integrate the Alexander Technique fundamentals and concepts into the narrative. For example, in the chapter "Hidden Causes of Repetitive Strain Injuries," the authors describe a case where a patient learns through conscious learning to overcome lower back pain through the Alexander Technique. In "Tools for Change," three guiding principles, all from the Alexander Technique, drive the authors prescription to combat RSI: (1) awareness of one's responses, (2) pause—withholding an automatic response (inhibition in the Alexander Technique), and (3) direction, that is, primary control. The remainder of the book describes the application of the authors' teachings of the Alexander Technique in basic movement activities, such as lying down, standing, walking, working at a desk and keyboarding, driving, and in jobs requiring use of the arms. They include appendixes for businesses who want to employ training solutions using this technique, an explanation of how the authors provide training and consulting, and a list of products.

Breathing Master Classes. **Malibu, Calif.: Windplayer Publications, 2002.**
This work is a collection of fourteen essays on breathing, therapies and techniques for better breathing, and the benefits of proper breathing techniques. Each essay is two pages in length and includes a biographical sketch of the essayist. One of the essays, written by Jessica Wolf, addresses how the Alexander Technique can improve breathing. Wolf is a certified Alexander Technique teacher and the "Art of Breathing" course director for Alexander teachers. She explains how the Alexander Technique teaches one to learn balance that restores natural

poise, which in turn increases the fluidity of the body and the breath. She describes a seven-point exercise to free up airflow and ease body tension, beginning with sitting comfortably with feet flat on the floor, then letting air out with a sigh, visualizing your breath rising upward, then repeating the cycles of the exercise and, finally, ending the exercise with a voice aloud "Aaah." Other essays include topics on deep breathing, strengthening the abdominal muscles, building stamina through exercise, calming performance anxiety, allergies and asthma, and several others.

Brennan, Richard. *The Alexander Technique: An Introductory Guide to Natural Poise for Health and Well-Being.* Shaftesbury, UK: Element, 1999.
Written for the novice, nontechnical person, this illustrated guide provides very practical advice on employing the Alexander Technique. A chapter is devoted to defining the Alexander Technique, and a chapter on the history of the technique is included. In these, as in all chapters, photo illustrations abound to demonstrate concepts and discussion points. Richard Brennan writes that the Alexander Technique has benefits for releasing tension, improving backaches, stiff neck or frozen shoulders, hypertension, asthma, arthritis, and depression, and includes brief explanations and several case studies. One chapter promotes "helping yourself" with an extensive discussion of unreliable sensory feelings, awareness of how simple body actions can be performed with greater ease and efficiency, and breathing. Practical exercises are also illustrated, such as using a book support in learning to build awareness while lying down. Brennan devotes a final chapter to a robust understanding of how to locate an Alexander Technique teacher and what to expect in an Alexander Technique session. He provides an excellent discussion of the short-term and long-term effects of Alexander Technique lessons.

———. *The Alexander Technique: Natural Poise for Health.* Shaftesbury, UK: Element, 1991.
This text is the earlier version of Brennan's work published in 1999 (see above), with almost the same title. The content is extremely similar and organized in much the same way, except this earlier edition has almost no illustrations and the few illustrations included are simple, black-and-white drawings. The coverage is structured the same as in his 1999 work, including chapters on what the Alexander Technique is and a history of the technique, plus chapters on the benefits of the technique, how it works, learning to apply the technique by oneself, and practical exercises. The practical exercises include the book support, which is better illustrated in his later version, lying down, squatting, and eyes. In the exercise on eyes, Brennan notes that Alexander believed our tensions are as a result of a lack of interest in the present, or the "mind-wandering habit." Eyes play an important role in keeping balance. Brennan describes use of the eyes and peripheral vision to stay in the present and help with mind wandering. A final chapter discusses reading other books, finding a teacher, issues in taking lessons, and the proper chair.

———. *The Alexander Technique Manual: A Step-by-Step Guide to Improve Breathing, Posture, and Well-Being.* **Boston: Journey Editions, 1996.**
This colorful text is designed as a practical guide to address the application of the Alexander Technique in reducing stress, in sports activities, and for pregnancy and childbirth. Early chapters describe the fundamentals of the Alexander Technique and how it is relevant to the average person. In the chapter on relevance to everyone, Brennan emphasizes that life is not an emergency as a discussion to direct the reader to learn the technique for stress reduction, through slowing down to allow our lives to unfold naturally. An extensive discussion on how children have natural poise and how natural maturity causes the spontaneity of these natural positions to disappear over time is included. This discussion is beautifully illustrated with color photographs. The chapter "Thinking in Activity" is a detailed discussion of primary directions to (1) allow the neck to be free, (2) allow the head to go forward and up, and (3) allow the back to lengthen and widen. Brennan uses these explanations in the context of basic activities, including standing, sitting, driving, walking, writing, working at a computer, reading, eating, and playing a musical instrument. One chapter illustrates practical exercises for reducing stress with full-page, color photographs, including directional graphics added to show proper alignment. In the chapter on sports, discussions on golf, soccer (labeled football as it is known in most of the world outside the United States), horse riding, cycling, running, pool (or billiards), and tennis are illustrated and explained. A chapter on pregnancy and childbirth also colorfully illustrates positions for physical activity and rest during pregnancy, coping with labor, and giving birth.

———. *The Alexander Technique Workbook: Your Personal Programme for Health, Poise, and Fitness.* **Shaftesbury, UK: Element, 1992.**
In sixteen chapters, Brennan provides a nontechnical, easy-to-read guide to the Alexander Technique. A history of the technique is provided as well as a good, commonsense explanation of seven reasons the Alexander Technique is needed by most everyone. In later chapters, simple but clear illustrations demonstrate concepts and applications of the technique. For example, poor and correct posture positions are shown with skeletal illustrations and with human form illustrations. The mechanics of movement are addressed in one chapter. Brennan also provides a chapter approach to faulty sensory perception, inhibition, direction, senses, habits and choices, and muscles and reflexes. Several case histories illustrate practical concerns of application. There is a brief bibliography, address list of organizations, and a useful index.

———. *Mind and Body Stress Relief with the Alexander Technique.* **London: Thorsons, 1998.**
Brennan has designed a practical guide to overcoming stress using the Alexander Technique. The bulk of this text explains five prime stress concerns and how the

technique can improve or eliminate the effects of these stress phenomena, including (1) physical effects of stress, (2) worry, (3) anxiety, (4) depression, and (5) stress and emotions. As an introduction to these concepts, he discusses how stress affects the quality of life and how to recognize it and its causes. He makes a cogent argument that the Alexander Technique is an antidote to stress. There is also a chapter on the history of the technique that defines the fundamental concepts. In his discussion of the physical effects of stress, he describes both the physical reactions of the body and stress and the manifestations stress can appear as, such as diseases, emotional problems, and pain. In discussing "worry," he emphasizes staying in the present, and in discussing "anxiety," he shows how the Alexander Technique can help through teaching one to let go. These chapters have practical exercises included, though the illustrations are sparse and simplistic. There is an excellent chapter on breathing. He notes that shallow breathing can exacerbate stress, worry, anxiety, and depression. Brennan concludes his work with an extensive list of testimonials on the benefits and validity of the technique.

Dachman, Kenneth A., and Joen Pritchard Kinnan. *The Self-Health Handbook: Low-Cost, Easy-to-Use Therapies from around the World.* New York: Facts on File, 1996.

The authors provide a directorylike listing of over fifty, well-established therapeutic techniques, applications, and therapies. Kenneth Dachman and Joen Kinnan state they have selected the therapies for inclusion based on two criteria: (1) they can be done by oneself (i.e., without a medical practitioner) and (2) are low cost. The therapies are intended to fit in the realm of holistic and alternative practices. The text is organized by entries in nine categories: (1) flowers, plants, and herbs; (2) healing through nature's elements; (3) eating for health; (4) exercising the body; (5) our healing hands; (6) the breath of life; (7) the mind as healer; (8) healing "arts" and hobbies; and (9) alternative healing systems and practices. The entry on the Alexander Technique is included in the "exercising the body" category along with aerobic exercise, callanetics, tai chi, and yoga. Each entry, including the one about the Alexander Technique, includes a brief definition, a list of physiological and psychological applications, collateral cross-therapies, contraindications, equipment and material needed, origin of the technique, instructions on how to use or apply the therapy or technique, a brief bibliography, and a resource groups list. For example, for the Alexander Technique, the collateral cross-therapy listed is "breathing exercises," and the contraindications suggest one should check with a health care provider before undertaking the technique for a physical ailment.

Forsstrom, Brita, and Mel Hampson. *The Alexander Technique for Pregnancy and Childbirth.* London: Gollancz, 1995.

Unlike Ilana Machover's book (see entry this text), Brita Forsstrom and Mel Hampson concentrate on pregnancy and childbirth with a briefer discussion of employment of the Alexander Technique in parenthood. Forsstrom is a mother and Hampson a midwife; they are trained Alexander Technique teachers. In addition to a good description of the theory of the Alexander Technique, the primary content of the text is divided between "The Alexander Way for Pregnancy" and "Labor and Birth." In discussions about pregnancy, the authors describe misuse, specifically how a pregnant woman compensates for the increased imbalance as the fetus grows, and then provide extensive descriptions of good use in pregnancy, such as use of the pelvis floor, abdominal muscles, standing, walking, sleeping, lifting, and relaxation. One chapter is devoted to breathing, especially an illustrated description of the whispered "ah," an exercise to encourage the release of tension in musculature restricting breathing, especially the jaw, throat, and neck. In the section on labor, the more common lying down positions for childbirth are eschewed for more active positions, both upright and crouching. Five basic positions are described and illustrated with black-and-white photographs: (1) the monkey, (2) lunge in labor, (3) squatting in labor, (4) kneeling in labor, and (5) all fours.

Garlick, David. *The Lost Sixth Sense: A Medical Scientist Looks at the Alexander Technique.* Kensington, Australia: Laboratory for Muscoskeletal and Postural Research, School of Physiology and Pharmacology, University of New South Wales, 1990.
David Garlick begins by noting that the anatomist, Charles Bell, identified a "sixth sense," beyond our normal senses of sight, smell, hearing, taste, and touch, which Bell said was the sense of limb and body position and movement. Garlick then argues that this sixth sense has become lost, or suppressed. His argument in his introduction is linked to his study of the Alexander Technique and describes the common occurrence of poor posture in society today. Garlick then goes on to describe and discuss four main Alexander Technique principles in the context of his medical understanding of Alexander's work. These include inhibition, directions, ends and means, and primary control. For example, in primary control, Garlick describes neck reflexes that are a result of inputs from neck muscle receptors combined with inputs from the organs of balance. Each of these four sections has simple but illustrative black-and-white diagrams of his main point or argument. The author then describes or defines several physiological mechanisms relevant to the Alexander Technique, including tendon receptors, skin and joint receptors, muscle fiber types, breathing, muscle contraction, trunk muscles and respiration, sense of effort, slow and quick movements, and sense of fatigue. Lastly, Garlick gives advice on finding a teacher and experiencing an Alexander Technique session.

Guide to Natural Healing. New Lanark, UK: Geddes & Grosset, 1997.
This is an encyclopedic guide to natural and alternative medicines and therapies. Entries are formatted as an encyclopedic narrative or essay, some with subheadings, several from one to four pages in length, and others as more involved essays. Over twenty-five main topics are provided, including the Alexander Tech-

nique. The Alexander Technique section is four pages in length with four subheadings structuring the narrative: (1) Breaking the Habit of Bad Posture, (2) Ar-
moring, (3) Correct Posture, and (4) Treatment. The first three describe Alexander's work in discovering the technique and the importance of consciously
learning to relearn good habits of posture and movement. The "treatment" section
takes up the bulk of the essay, three pages, and describes the fundamentals of the
technique, using simple graphic illustrations of standing, sitting, and writing.
Some of the other healing therapies included in the book are acupuncture, polarity therapy, yoga, reflexology, Reiki, hypnotherapy, spiritual healing, aromatherapy, and herbal and essential oils remedies.

**Herring, Marq A., and Molly Manning Roberts, eds. *Blackwell Comple-
mentary and Alternative Medicine: Fast Facts for Medical Practice.*
Malden, Mass.: Blackwell, 2002.**
Written for professionals in health-related fields, the authors describe the value
and potential concerns of complementary and alternative medicines (CAM), including the significance of CAM in health care; guidelines for advising patients
about CAM; political and economic issues in CAM; and psychoneuroimmunol-
ogy (PNI), as a link to holism, or the concept of an individual's health as "unique
to one's constitution and attitudes." The authors argue that CAM is important to
the medical provider because people are choosing both traditional (or allopathic)
medicine and CAM therapies and techniques, not always keeping medical practitioners informed of their use of these therapies so that medical professionals are
required to learn more about integrating them into a total health prescription. After the chapters that discuss CAM in general, thirteen therapies and techniques are
described, including the Alexander Technique (in a chapter with the Feldenkrais
Method), acupuncture, hypnosis, homeopathy, massage therapy, music therapy,
Reiki, tai chi, and others. In the chapter on the Alexander Technique and
Feldenkrais, the technique is described with encyclopedic subcategories on how
it is used, what the indications for use are, expected outcomes, how the technique
works, scientific evidence of its validity as a therapy, and issues of certification
and licensure. A case study also illustrates a practical application.

**Macdonald, Glynn. *The Complete Illustrated Guide to Alexander Technique:
A Practical Program for Health, Poise, and Fitness.* Shaftesbury, UK: Element,
1998.**

**———. *Natural Ways to Health, Alexander Technique: A Practical Program
for Health, Poise, and Fitness.* Alexandria, Va.: TimeLife Books, 1998.**
These two books by Glynn Macdonald are exact in every way except for
the publisher. *The Complete Illustrated Guide to Alexander Technique* is the
British publication of the TimeLife series title. Much of these two books
are designed in the same manner as the TimeLife publishing library. Created
for the average consumer, the emphasis is on many colorful illustrations and

photographs and a layout designed to compartmentalize information with the use of column dividers and efficient use of white space. The book does include copious amounts of relevant information divided into five main sections: (1) Man's Supreme Inheritance (the history of the technique and its development); (2) The Use of the Self (practical experience, physiological information, and the procedures of Raymond Dart; (3) Constructive Conscious Control (the three areas of application being education, sports and recreation, and the performing arts); (4) The Universal Constant in Living (where self-learning plays a significant role); and (5) Resources, including a glossary, readings list, and useful addresses. The illustrations dominate the text but are clear, attractive, and informative.

MacDonnell, Michele. *Alexander Technique for Health and Well-Being.* London: Southwater, 1999.
Michele MacDonnell's work is designed to be a layperson's guide to specific health practices guided by the Alexander Technique. The book is lushly illustrated with color photographs on every page. Each health practice or activity is described and illustrated on two facing pages. The first ten pages provide a brief history of the Alexander Technique and the most fundamental concepts of primary control, means-whereby, sensory appreciation or awareness, and natural poise (a discussion of how children have natural posture that is often lost by people as they grow up). The bulk of the book is formatted with specific topics, such as kneeling, use of the eyes, sitting, standing, tiptoes, reaching and handling, the "monkey" or bending, "lunge monkey," squatting, walking, lifting, carrying, use of a telephone, driving, work at a computer, and others. All explanations are concise and fully illustrated.

Machover, Ilana, Angela Drake, and Jonathan Drake. *The Alexander Technique Birth Book: A Guide to Better Pregnancy, Natural Childbirth, and Parenthood.* New York: Sterling Publishing, 1993.
The authors have written a guide about how beneficial the Alexander Technique is to the preparation for pregnancy and childbirth, and for physical health during the early stages of parenthood. Ilana Machover is an Alexander Technique teacher and an advanced teacher for Britain's National Childbirth Trust. Angela and Jonathan Drake are parents of three children and have used the Alexander Technique in childbirth and parenting. Jonathan is the author of two known texts on the Alexander Technique. This guide shows how to cope effectively with the demands of feeding and lifting, and carrying a baby. Substantial advice is given on early pregnancy first, then late pregnancy. For example, bending to tie a shoe while pregnant is an exercise called "the monkey," with a full explanation accompanied by an illustration and black-and-white photographs to show how leverage in the legs improves standing and bending. Movements such as lying down, kneeling, and crawling are illustrated similarly in the later pregnancy chapter. An extensive discussion on giving birth is provided, complete with instruc-

tions on coping with labor pains, breathing naturally, and positioning to give birth, including kneeling on all fours for birthing.

Stevens, Christopher, ed. *The F. M. Alexander Technique: Medical and Physiological Aspects.* 2nd ed. Devon, UK: Author, 1994.
This work constitutes the proceedings of the F. M. Alexander Technique: Medical and Physiological Aspects Conference, held at Aalborg Folk University in Denmark on November 29, 1987. The inside cover indicates a one-day conference that included five conference papers, a documentary film *Posture and Pain*, and a session of demonstrations of the Alexander Technique. This publication reproduces the five conference papers. Christopher Stevens's paper provides an overview of research on the Alexander Technique, especially a discussion of Wilfred Barlow's work with army recruits, 40 students from the Royal College of Music, and 112 female physical education teachers, and Frank Pierce Jones's study with X-ray photographs. Michael Nielsen's paper discusses stress among professional musicians, in a report on an experiment using three methods of reducing stress, including the Alexander Technique, exercise, and use of beta-blockers. In Kathleen Ballard's paper, muscle spindles are described and discussed, complete with diagrams, as a broader discussion of their relevance to the Alexander Technique. Finn Bejsen-Moller's paper describes elastic tissues and their role in movement, with particular attention to the Alexander Technique and positioning of the spine. Lastly, David Gorman describes some psychophysical principles in functional anatomy.

————. *Towards a Physiology of the F. M. Alexander Technique: A Record of Work in Progress.* London: Distributed by STAT Books, 1995.
Stevens, a physicist and professor of anatomy, is a trained Alexander Technique teacher who has conducted a number of scientific research projects on the Alexander Technique. In this book, he describes and discusses his research and that of a significant body of other research studies. He begins with a brief coverage of early scientific opinion and the experimental studies by Wilfred Barlow and Frank Pierce Jones. Stevens performed seven different experiments and other research projects, including three experiments on the sit-to-stand movement, two experiments of height and shoulder width changes, and a study of stress-related increase in blood pressure. Each of the seven studies is thoroughly explained, complete with illustrations and diagrams. For example, in his experiment on the sit-to-stand movement, he examined three dimensions: head displacement, head velocities, and force platform. Diagrams illustrating these include a path diagram of head movement, a scale measurement of horizontal anteroposterior velocity of the head, and a scale of vertical forces from the seat and feet. Each experiment includes a description of methodology and the results. Stevens then discusses the findings of Alexander research in light of current scientific concepts of proprioception, stretch reflex, elasticity, muscle, the brain, touch, responses to overbalancing and movement, the startle pattern, and eye, labyrinth, and neck reflexes.

Tinbergen, Nikolaas. *Ethology and Stress Diseases: An Examination of the Alexander Technique.* **Champaign, Ill.: NASTAT (North American Society of Teachers of the Alexander Technique), 1974.**

This brief, four-page publication is the complete text of Nikolaas Tinbergen's Nobel Prize for Medicine acceptance speech. Tinbergen was awarded the 1973 Nobel for Medicine for "discoveries in the field of the organization and occurrence of individual and social behavioral patterns" in the animal world. Tinbergen was one of the founders of the field of ethology, the branch of biology that studies animal behavior. Half of his Nobel acceptance speech was devoted to the Alexander Technique because of the benefits he and his wife enjoyed from the technique. Fully half of his discussion of the Alexander Technique is a personal anecdote of his experience with his own exploration and lessons. He makes a cogent argument for the efficacy of the technique as well, stating, "There is no doubt that it often does have profound and beneficial effects and . . . both in the mental and somatic sphere." He notes that, in the field of ethology, the recent discovery of the concept of reafference (that the correct performance of the many movements is checked by the brain) makes the Alexander Technique more understandable and more plausible.

ARTICLES

Abenhaim, Lucien, et al. "Role of Activity in the Therapeutic Management of Back Pain: Report of the International Paris Task Force on Back Pain." *SPINE: The International Journal for the Study of the Spine* **25, no. 45, supplement (February 15, 2000): 15–33S.**

This article is a meta-analysis review of significant research literature and other publications on the role of physical activities as therapy for low back pain. This analysis is grouped into broad categories, including research on (1) occupational activity, (2) mobility and daily living activity, and (3) recreational and sports-related activities, including exercise. Each broad category defines and reviews the issues affecting therapies for low back pain, describes the research findings for use of these activities as therapies, and then makes recommendations on the value of that activity as therapy for back pain. For example, research on bed rest as an issue of mobility and daily living was analyzed, and this study found that bed rest does not improve on back pain in significant ways. In the category on "exercise," the Alexander Technique is defined briefly and mentioned as a nontraditional form of exercise-related therapy. Though the authors produce a statistical analysis of their metadata research on articles reporting exercise as a therapy for low back pain, the research on the Alexander Technique is not specifically analyzed.

Austin, J. H., and P. Ausubel. "Enhanced Respiratory Muscular Function in Normal Adults after Lessons in Proprioceptive Musculoskeletal Education without Exercises." *Chest* **102, no. 2 (August 1992): 486–90.**

The authors conducted a clinical trial of the enhanced ease of breathing through the application of the Alexander Technique. An experimental and control group of ten healthy adult subjects each were created, matched for age, gender, height, and weight. The experimental group received twenty Alexander Technique lessons at weekly intervals. Before and after each lesson, all subjects were given spirometric tests, including maximum static mouth pressures. The results showed that the experimental group showed significant increases on four parameters of the test, while the control group did not record any significant changes. The authors concluded that the Alexander Technique may enhance respiratory functions in normal adults.

Barnet, Ellen Gribben. "Move Away from the Pain: Try 'Posture Rehab' with the Alexander Technique." *Prevention* **54 (June 2002): 85.**
This short article relates the author's personal experience with back pain caused by a car accident. On the advice of a medical professional, she found the benefits of the Alexander Technique. The author does not explain the method in any way but reports excellent success with retraining her body for better posture. She provides the contact information for the American Society for the Alexander Technique to locate a teacher.

Batson, Glenna. "Conscious Use of the Human Body in Movement: The Peripheral Neuro-anatomic Basis of the Alexander Technique." *Medical Problems of Performing Artists* **11, no. 1 (March 1996): 3–12.**
The author "discusses the peripheral neuro-anatomic basis for the Alexander Technique: the role played by the body's proprioceptors (the peri- and intra-articular neural afferents) in movement organization." Proprioceptive training, which is a form of reeducation used in orthopedic and sports medicine rehabilitation, is compared and contrasted with the Alexander Technique principles in depth. Glenna Batson argues that Alexander must have known of the study of proprioception, though he never mentions it, because of the significant parallels in Alexander's method of self-teaching approach to posture and movement at the exact time scientific theories on proprioception were being developed. For example, Alexander focused on methods of releasing tension patterns in the neck just when neurophysiologists discovered massive numbers of muscle spindles in the cervical musculature. Batson also describes the history of proprioception, which in today's connotation relates just to posture and position, and kinesthesia, which concerns a sense of movement. The scientific work in this field involves the study of various afferent neurons called "mechanoreceptors" in and around the joint capsules, which act as transducers, converting a specific physical stimulus into a neural pulse. Batson explains how Alexander's work has transformed human movement science from the theory that individual receptors act as regulators of proprioception and movement to a theory centered in a systems approach to motor control and motor learning.

Begley, Sharon. "Alternative Medicine: A Cure for What Ails Us?" *American Health* **11, no. 3 (April 1992): 38–46.**
This informative article in a popular health magazine discusses the arguments for and against alternative medicines and therapies, then describes, briefly, eleven of

these, including the Alexander Technique, acupuncture, biofeedback, hypnosis, osteopathy, chiropractic, Hellerwork, reflexology, therapeutic touch, aromatherapy, and naturopaths. The author describes why people choose alternatives, including statistics on how many people report considering these therapies and other data. The primary reasons stated are a desire to take more of an active role in their health and therapy and the willingness to enhance traditional medicine. The skepticism and arguments against alternative therapies within the medical profession is also discussed. The Alexander Technique is described in a brief paragraph.

Britton, A. G. "Working Out the Invisible Self." *American Health* **8, no. 2 (March 1989): 68–74.**
A. G. Britton describes the trend in aerobic exercise to create a mind-body work in dance exercise, especially. She discusses the International Dance Exercise Association's (IDEA) concept of "integration," or, in other words, mind-body work and how dance exercise instructors now emphasize a workout that brings the mind and spirit into the exercise. Some specific examples are described in some depth, including use of visual imagery, proprioceptive neuromuscular facilitation (PNF) in aerobics, and Yokibics (aerobic exercise that combines yoga techniques). Britton clearly attributes this phenomenon to the influence of the Alexander Technique and other mind-body techniques but does not discuss the Alexander Technique at any length.

Brockbank, Nancy. "Alexander Self-help." *Positive Health* **60 (January 2001): 51–52.**
The author makes a cogent argument that most of us find it difficult to teach ourselves the Alexander Technique because having a faulty sense of ourselves makes change difficult. She suggests there are alternative ways to find self-help with the technique. First, two steps are described to develop a proper mindset, including (1) becoming fully engaged in what we are doing and the way it is done, and (2) recognizing what we are doing and what is being done wrong. To this end, she details an exercise to test what is being done. This begins with instructions to place the palm of the hand on the back of the neck and then trying to stand, looking for what the neck muscles do (tension and tightening). A variation, placing one hand on the back of the head and one on the forehead, is also described. Additional discussions describe ways Alexander encouraged awareness.

Cacciatore, Timothy W., Fay B. Horak, and Sharon M. Henry. "Improvement in Automatic Postural Coordination following Alexander Technique Lessons in a Person with Low Back Pain." *Physical Therapy* **85, no. 6 (June 2005): 565–78.**
The authors begin with the concept that a relationship between back pain and abnormal postural coordination is not clearly understood or defined. They begin by describing the Alexander Technique as a therapy to improve postural coordination by

using conscious processes to change how a person automatically moves and maintains posture or coordination of posture, and muscular activity. They note evidence that shows the Alexander Technique can reduce low back pain. Using a case study, the authors describe the use of the technique with a client, a forty-nine-year-old woman with a twenty-five-year history of left-sided, idiopathic, lumbrosacral back pain. A force plate during horizontal platform translations was used to measure automatic postural coordination and one-legged standing. Tests of the client's postural coordination and back pain were taken for four months prior to Alexander Technique lessons and three months after lessons concluded. The authors found that the client had laterally asymmetric automatic postural responses to translations prior to the lessons but that the magnitude and asymmetry of her responses and balance improved after the lessons. Additionally, she experienced reduced low back pain.

Dennis, J., and C. Cates. "Alexander Technique for Chronic Asthma." *Cochrane Database System Review* 2 (2000): CD000995.
The authors report a database search and review to locate research on the application of the Alexander Technique as an asthma therapy or complementary and alternative medicine strategy in improving asthma conditions. They report their search sought research using randomized controlled trials comparing the treatment with either another intervention or no intervention. Their search found no evidence of such research, and the authors concluded that, without this research evidence, Alexander Technique practitioners cannot claim the technique aids in improving chronic asthma.

Dennis, R. J. "Functional Reach Improvement in Normal, Older Women after Alexander Technique Instruction." *Journal of Gerontology: A Biological Science/Medical Science* 54, no. 1 (January 1999): M8–11.
The author studied a possible relationship between "functional reach" and the Alexander Technique. Functional reach is a clinical measure of balance. For this research, three groups of women over the age of sixty-five were formed: (1) a pilot group, (2) an experimental group, and (3) a control group. An additional control group of older men was also formed. The pilot and experimental groups were given eight, one-hour sessions of the Alexander Technique at two-week intervals. Pretests and posttests were administered to measure functional reach. Dennis found that the Alexander Technique contributed to a significant improvement in functional reach in both the pilot and experimental groups. The experimental group was retested one month after the posttest and showed signs of slightly decreased functional reach. Both groups were also given a four-item qualitative questionnaire to measure an overall positive response to Alexander Technique instruction.

Dranov, Paula. "Alternatives: Does Bodywork Work?" *Health* 15, no. 3 (April 2001): 80–83.
In her featured column on alternative therapies, Paula Dranov argues that body techniques, explained in this article, can aid in improving posture and awkward

movements, and that this can lead to improved body health. She mentions that research on how effective these techniques are is sparse. Her intent is to aid readers in choosing which technique is appropriate for them. Five techniques are described in the following format: (1) a paragraph on the development of the
technique, (2) a paragraph on a "typical visit," and (3) a brief statement on cost
and how to locate a teacher. The five techniques include (1) the Alexander Technique, (2) Feldenkrais, (3) the Trager Approach, (4) Aston-Patterning, and (5)
Hellerwork. For a typical visit to an Alexander Technique teacher, Dranov notes
that the teacher will watch the way you carry yourself and offer suggestions and
guide your limbs as you move. Dranov states that the Alexander Technique promotes getting the head, neck, and spine into proper alignment through "unlearning" poor posture habits.

Dworkin, Norine. "Besting Bad Backs." *Vegetarian Times* **252 (August 1998): 60–61.**
Norine Dworkin briefly argues that eating a vegetarian diet, exercise, and the
right supplements can maintain back health. She then lists fifteen therapies or
techniques she notes can ease back pain should it occur. Those mentioned include
the Alexander Technique, acupuncture, chiropractic, Feldenkrais, magnet therapy, reflexology, Rolfing, the Trager Approach, yoga, and others. Each entry includes a very brief annotation that lists the core purpose of the technique. For the
Alexander Technique, Dworkin notes that the technique seeks to disrupt the
body's habitual holding and movement postures.

Elkayam, O., E. Avrahami, and M. Yaron. "The Lack of Prognostic Value of Computerized Tomography Imaging Examinations in Patients with Chronic Non-progressive Back Pain." *Rheumatology International* **16, no. 1 (1996): 19–21.**
The authors conducted a clinical study of the prognostic value of a computerized
tomography (CT) scan on seventy-three patients with chronic, nonprogressive
back pain in the lumbar region. Each patient was given an examination and spinal
scan before rehabilitation therapies were applied. All patients then received four
weeks of therapies from a multidisciplinary approach, including the Alexander
Technique, acupuncture, manipulation, and psychological intervention, in addition to the treatment by a rheumatologist. Three separate postexperimental groups
then received a scan based on the CT examination results. The authors concluded
that these procedures did not significantly contribute to a prognosis.

Elkayam, O., et al. "Multidisciplinary Approach to Chronic Back Pain: Prognostic Elements of the Outcome." *Clinical Experimental Rheumatology* **14, no. 3 (May/June 1996): 281–88.**
The authors sought to examine if a multidisciplinary approach to back pain ther-
apy improved patients' health. Using a treatment and control group, with a total
of sixty-seven patients who experienced back pain of three months or more, a

plan to administer a comprehensive, four-week program was created. Patients received application or treatment in the Alexander Technique, back schooling, acupuncture, chiropractic, and psychological intervention, and with a pain specialist. A sociodemographic questionnaire and a psychological evaluation using a questionnaire and an interview were used as the pretest and to group the participants based on three criteria: (1) predominance of psychological factors, (2) secondary pain, and (3) personality features. The patient evaluation was administered again as the posttest. The results showed that this multidisciplinary approach significantly improved the patients' pain rating, pain frequency, and analgesic drug consumption. Psychological factors were also correlated and showed a satisfactory performance for psychological factors and family support, but a poor outcome was correlated to factors including divorce, unemployment, and personality disorders.

Gilman, Marina, and J. Scott Yarass. "Stuttering and Relaxation: Applications for Somatic Education in Stuttering Treatment." *Journal of Fluency Disorders* 25, no. 1 (Spring 2000): 59–76.
The authors pose the view that relaxation techniques can be an integral part of therapeutic treatment of stuttering disorders. They begin with a literature review of the link between relaxation techniques and stuttering treatment and a history of this approach. They found that relaxation as a therapeutic approach was common from the nineteenth century until within the past thirty years but that it fell out of favor as a therapy due to the belief that "the sensation of being relaxed is difficult to generalize and so has limited efficacy outside the treatment environment." The authors then propose that somatic education in the form of three techniques—the Alexander Technique, Rolfing, and Feldenkrais—leads them to a new definition of relaxation, that is, "Relaxation is a state of being or feeling, resulting from increased stability of the neuro-muscular systems and the concomitant coordination of muscles through the entire body. Ease of movement . . . is the result of the smooth transition from states of instability to stability." The authors then describe the specific principles of the Alexander Technique, Rolfing, and Feldenkrais and how they related to relaxation in the treatment of stuttering. They also discuss implications for research on this topic.

Jamil, Tanvir. "Posture Therapies: Guide to Complementary Therapies." *Pulse* 63, no. 19 (May 12, 2003): 76.
This article discusses the evidence base for the Alexander Technique and Feldenkrais. Tanvir Jamil notes that these are the two main forms of posture therapy, then briefly describes how each technique can benefit the individual. Three research studies are then listed with an annotation describing their primary findings. Jamil also provides a table listing the pros and cons, with the pros as (1) safe, (2) often organized by local organizations, and (3) books and videos readily available; and cons as (1) cost, (2) time, and (3) difficulty in learning.

Karlson, Amy Elizabeth. "In Fine Form." *Vegetarian Times* **302 (October 2002): 107–12.**

Amy Karlson discusses how posture plays a significant role in one's health. She describes how posture is defined by medical professionals, and she explains "proper position." She makes a case that many people have poor posture due to habits from sitting too much and exercising too little, as well as habits of poor positioning. She notes that an ideal posture is when the head is resting directly over your shoulders in the body's center of gravity. The basics of standing, sitting, and sleeping are described. None of these discussions mention or attribute them to the Alexander Technique. Additionally, Karlson argues that diet and obesity also play a role in body stress and poor posture. Following this general discussion of posture, the author describes five techniques for body work and better posture, including (1) the Alexander Technique, (2) yoga, (3) chiropractic, (4) acupuncture, and (5) massage. The discussion of the Alexander Technique is a very brief description of the core purpose of teaching people to properly align the head, neck, and torso. The remaining discussion explains some stretching exercises.

Kotzsch, Ronald. "The Alexander Technique: An Effective Therapy for Medical Problems?" *East West Journal* **20, no. 1 (October 1990): 34–42.**

Ronald Kotzsch uses numerous interviews with Alexander Technique teachers to explain the appeal of the technique. He begins by relating his sense of being underwhelmed by his own first lesson, having assumed that there would be more exercise. His interview with Yehuda Kuperman, an Alexander Technique teacher in Basel, Switzerland, confirms this feeling as Kuperman reported a similar experience. Yet, both soon realized that they learned something about themselves from their first lesson. Kuperman noted it gave him a positive sense of himself. Kotzsch explains that the technique helps people gain a sense of a balanced body, with increased sense of efficiency and ease. He describes the history and development of the Alexander Technique, including a discussion of how Alexander was considered a kind of medical quack by many physicians for a time. Kotzsch describes working with over twenty Alexander Technique teachers. He found that many do not regard the Alexander Technique as therapy but rather consider it lessons in use of the self and manipulative body work. He interviewed Antje Hindemann and Deborah Caplan, both Alexander Technique teachers. Caplan wrote *Back Trouble: A New Approach to Prevention and Recovery Based on the Alexander Technique* and is the daughter of one of the first Alexander Technique teachers in America. Both describe use of the body as crucial to the technique. Hindemann notes that her measure of success is the student's development of proper use. Caplan states that the concept of use is basic to the technique's understanding of the cause of musculoskeletal problems. Kotzsch also describes teacher training programs in America, provides a brief description of basic aspects of a typical lesson, including costs, and provides contact information for NASTAT (the North American Society of Teachers of the Alexander Technique) and STAT

(Society of Teachers of the Alexander Technique—the British Alexander Technique organization).

Kristl, Margaret. "The Alexander Technique as a Management Tool of a Connective Tissue Disorder." *Journal of Bodywork and Management Therapies* 5, no. 3 (July 2001): 181–90.
The author describes the basics of Marfan syndrome, a genetic disorder of the connective tissue throughout the body. She defines the Alexander Technique as an aid to improving the Marfan syndrome by promoting the psychophysical unity of the individual. Margaret Kristl makes a cogent argument that the Alexander Technique allows people to improve their health through the use of self-observation and attention to everyday life activities. She also notes that the Alexander Technique has a direct application to other manifestations of the Marfan syndrome such as scoliosis, back pain, and trauma damage to vocal cords due to surgery.

Machover, Ilana. "Turn, Baby, Turn." *Midwives* 108, no. 1295 (December 1995): 389–91.
Ilana Machover describes a series of steps that can be taken to improve the chances that a breech baby will turn into a normal position for birth; she developed these steps from her work as an Alexander Technique instructor. She begins by describing the issues and concerns regarding breech babies, including statistics on the number of breech babies, traditional approaches to get the baby to turn, and the generally poor state of communication interaction between breech baby mothers and medical personnel. She describes discovering the Elkins knee-chest position and a study that seemed to show greater success when women rolled onto their hands and knees after the procedure. Machover argues that the Alexander Technique can inform this method and improve breech baby repositioning. She lists a step-by-step guide to her technique.

Maitland, Sheila, Roger Horner, and Mark Burton. "An Exploration of the Application of the Alexander Technique for People with Learning Disabilities." *British Journal of Learning Disabilities* 24, no. 2 (1996): 70–76.
The authors conducted a study of introducing Alexander Technique lessons to learning disabled individuals. Eight people with varying degrees of learning disabilities, some with limited communication skills, were provided hands-on instruction, seeking to aid in posture, spasticity, and anxiety. Problems encountered are discussed as well as an explanation of the Alexander Technique and its fundamentals. The authors concluded that it may have benefits in this context but that more research is needed.

Mandelbaum-Schmid, Judith. "Natural Pain Killers: Safe, Alternative Treatment for Backaches, Headaches, PMS, and More." *McCall's* 125, no. 12 (September 1998): 94–95.
The author of the popular women's journal article describes alternative therapies as "becoming mainstream." She quotes a Stanford University study that found

people seek alternative therapies not as a rejection of medical treatment but because they recognize that true healing involves the entire self: mind, body, and spirit. The bulk of the article is set in sections, each dealing with a condition for which one or more therapies offers help. These conditions include PMS, tension headache, backache, the common cold, menstrual cramps, and tension. The Alexander Technique is only discussed in the "backache" paragraphs. The article does not explain the technique at all but advises the reader to seek lessons. It does state that it is a hands-on method to release neck muscles and to hold the head in a more relaxed manner.

Mehling, Wolf E., Zelda DiBlasi, and Frederick Hecht. "Bias Control in Trials of Bodywork: A Review of Methodological Issues." *Journal of Alternative and Complementary Medicine* **11, no. 2 (April 2005): 333–42.**
The authors searched PubMed and EMBASE electronic databases for medical literature to review and summarize the methodological challenges in clinical trials of body-work or hands-on mind-body therapies such as Feldenkrais, Alexander Technique, Trager Approach, Eutony, Body Awareness Therapy, Breath Therapy, and Rolfing. Published bibliographies were also examined for this research. Published clinical studies of individual hands-on approaches were also included if they focused on body awareness and were not based on technical devices. In their review, fifty-three studies were identified with twenty exhibiting a complete set of inclusion criteria. The authors found that blind subject methodology was not used with any student; however, five used an alternative treatment while blinding participants to differential investigator expectations of efficacy. Furthermore, they discovered that a credible placebo intervention was not used in any of the studies. Also, they could not identify any study that reported patient expectations, which is common in other studies of alternative therapies and medicines. The authors conclude with suggestions for minimizing investigator and therapist bias and bias from differential patient expectations.

Prentice, C., A. M. Canty, and I. Janowitz. "Back School Programs: The Pregnant Patient and Her Partner." *Occupational Medicine* **7, no. 1 (January–March 1992): 77–85.**
The authors promote patient education for pregnant women and their partners, emphasizing that pregnancy needs three months prior to conception (when planning a pregnancy) to change diets and exercise routines for an overall health regimen. In this article, the authors note that the Alexander Technique is a valuable approach for pregnant women to develop posture and body mechanics, and improve use of the body. They see this as enabling patients to learn to help themselves to reduce long-term therapy. They also believe there is a need to inform health care professionals about the benefits of the Alexander Technique.

Rhodes, Maura. "Wind Down Workout." *Health* **21 (February 1989): 50–51.**
This short article includes one page of text and one page with a photoset illustrating the workout. The author is a "movement consultant" and certified Alexan-

der Technique teacher. She promotes the technique as a mind-body method for becoming aware of and changing habits that can cause tension and pain. The workout is described in eleven steps. These are very specific movements beginning with "lie on back, feet flat, fingertips resting on hip joints" to "reach with right arm to lead right side of body back onto bed."

Ribeaux, P., and M. Spence. "CAM Evaluation: What Are the Research Questions?" *Complementary Therapies in Medicine* 9 (2001): 188–93.
CAM therapies (complementary and alternative medicines) are often evaluated for their effectiveness and validity before identification of the relevant research questions. Typical CAM therapies included in these authors' discussions include the Alexander Technique, reflexology, chiropractic, acupuncture, aromatherapy, osteopathy, spiritual healing, yoga, and dance movement therapy, among others. The authors note that traditional research on medicines and therapies utilize the random controlled trial, which requires isolating extraneous factors. This method of research is seen as inappropriate for the more holistic therapies because (1) the core factor or active ingredient of a therapy changes from patient to patient and (2) the form measurement omits important aspects of a holistic skill. The authors provide their taxonomy of holistic therapies, listing the Alexander Technique, bioenergetic therapy, yoga, and dance movement therapy as the most holistic, and herbal medicine, osteopathy, chiropractic, and reflexology as the least holistic. Therapies that are the least holistic are able to utilize traditional research, that is, the randomized controlled trial, more readily, while this form of research is less of a fit for the most holistic types. From this discussion, they go on to suggest ways of seeking research questions when formulating assessment methods of these therapies.

Smith, Derek. "Developing the Self as a Therapeutic Tool." *Australian Nursing Journal* 10, no. 10 (May 2003): 33.
Derek Smith describes a report from a popular weekly magazine on nurse-patient relationships, showing strong, interpersonal skills are responsible for effective nursing practice. However, Smith argues that developing an awareness of the self by nurses in order to meet the needs of their patients is necessary. Most approaches to becoming aware of the self, however, focus on psychological aspects. Smith makes a cogent case that a more holistic approach for a greater psychophysical awareness is needed. He gives a brief history of the Alexander Technique, then explains how the Alexander Technique provides strategies and process to become more efficient through development of awareness and use of the self.

———. "Prevention Is Better than Cure." *Australian Nursing Journal* 7, no. 8 (March 2000): 30.
Smith briefly discusses an Australian study of health and community services workers that found that 14 percent of all workers' compensation claims for body stress came from this sector and that preventing this with training on the proper

way to lift objects was the best approach. A brief explanation of the Alexander
Technique is used to promote the technique as a form of prevention in these cases.

Stallibrass, Chloe. "An Evaluation of the Alexander Technique for the Management of Disability in Parkinson's Disease: A Preliminary Study." *Clinical Rehabilitation* **11, no. 1 (February 1997): 8–12.**
A pilot study was developed to test the therapeutic effect of Alexander Technique
lessons on Parkinson's disease patients. Seven individuals with the disease were
recruited who exhibited both idiopathic symptoms of the disease and feelings of
depression. Participants received four self-report questionnaires, one set before
Alexander Technique lessons and the remaining after the lessons were completed.
Participants received twelve lessons in the Alexander Technique. Outcome measures used were the Beck Depression Inventory and three self-report questionnaires on daily life, body concept, and social functioning disability. The study
found that the subjects who received the Alexander Technique were significantly
less depressed, with a margin of error of approximately 5 percent, as well as significantly more positive body concept and less difficulty in performing daily tasks.

Stallibrass, Chloe, and Mel Hampson. "The Alexander Technique: Its Application in Midwifery and the Results of Preliminary Research into Parkinson's." *Complementary Therapies in Nursing and Midwifery* **7 (2001): 13–18.**
The authors begin with the premise that the Alexander Technique is a method for
informed self-observation to recognize habitual patterns of misuse and, as a result, a method of self-help. However, they recognize the need for proper hands-on instruction to reach the point of self-help. A detailed explanation of the fundamentals is provided including its origins, primary control, the psychophysical
unity, use of the self, and what a typical Alexander Technique lesson is like. Recent research into the efficacy of the technique is also described. In the final two
sections of the article, the authors describe applications of the Alexander Technique for pregnancy and childbirth, and they report the preliminary results of a
randomized control trial of use of the Alexander Technique for alleviating symptoms of Parkinson's disease.

Stallibrass, Chloe, P. Sissions, and C. Chalmers. "Randomized Controlled Trial of the Alexander Technique for Idiopathic Parkinson's Diseases." *Clinical Rehabilitation* **16, no. 7 (November 1, 2002): 695–708.**
The authors conducted a pilot study in 1997 using the Alexander Technique in
conjunction with a drug therapy to determine the benefits of the Alexander Technique with Parkinson's disease. That study indicated further study would be
promising if administered with a larger group. The article reports the results of
the second, larger effort. The researchers used a larger sample, ninety-three in all,
of Parkinson's disease patients using an experimental group and two control
groups, with randomized assignment to all three groups. The experimental group
received twenty-four Alexander Technique lessons. One control group received

twenty-four sessions of massage therapy. The outcome measures given as a pretest and posttest were the Self-Assessment Parkinson's Disease Disability Scale (SPDDS), Beck Depression Inventory, and an attitudes to self scale. The results of the study showed that the Alexander Technique group improved compared with the control group receiving no intervention, both at the best and worse times of the day, and also showed less signs of depression, as measured on the Beck Depression Inventory. The authors concluded that Alexander Technique lessons can lead to sustained benefits for Parkinson's disease patients.

Stedman, Nancy. "Getting Straight." *Health* **17 (November 1985): 65–67.**
The author begins by describing herself as always having a sense of limberness, able to contort her body in all manner and ways from a very young age. However, by her thirties, she felt a loss of balance. After hearing about the Alexander Technique, she began lessons to relieve lower back tension and to regain this sense of balance. She states there are two main principles: (1) inhibiting unnecessary muscle movement and (2) carrying the head and body in an upward direction. She tells her readers that Alexander Technique lessons are not a simple solution. She found two obstacles to overcome: (1) the length of time to see real change, generally three to six months, and (2) overcoming the psychological inhibition used to control how we use our body. Nancy Stedman recounts a very lengthy description of her lessons with Ann Rodiger, an Alexander Technique teacher in Manhattan. She provides a robust description of the lesson while lying down on a table and indicates that this position gave her a great deal of release from tension.

Stocker, Sharon. "Move Away from Pain." *Prevention* **54, no. 6 (June 2002): 85.**
A brief article that relates the benefit gained by Ellen Bornet, who underwent Alexander Technique instruction after a car accident severely damaged her neck, back, knees, and jaw. After more traditional therapies were tried, a neurologist recommended the Alexander Technique. The author describes the basic methods used in a typical therapy session and the patient's success.

Sullivan, Karin Horgan. "Perfect Posture." *Vegetarian Times* **257 (January 1999): 64–68.**
Karin Sullivan discusses posture as important to health and describes poor posture as including thrusting your head forward and excessive arching of your lower back. She notes that stiffening to a military-style "stand at attention" also is a poor choice because it can stiffen the neck, lock breathing, and arch the back. Four techniques for better posture are then described, including (1) the Alexander Technique, (2) chiropractic, (3) Rolfing, and (4) yoga. In discussing the Alexander Technique, Sullivan briefly describes a typical lesson as taught one-on-one in thirty minutes to an hour with a minimum of ten sessions recommended. In the lesson, the teacher guides you through individual movement patterns. An exercise to lengthen the spine and release muscle tension is then explained. The article

also includes an "editor's pick" section that lists products that can be purchased for stretching, sitting right, and back rest, including a "lying down on the back bridge" to lengthen the spine and expand the chest, shoulder, and rib cage, as well as a price list and vendor contacts.

Trevelyan, Joanna. "Alexander Technique." *Nursing Times* **89, no. 49 (December 8, 1993): 50–52.**
The author describes the Alexander Technique as a psychophysical educational method to aid individuals in building poise and balance in movement and attitude. She explains the essentials of the instruction as a one-on-one set of lessons, using words and gentle touch, to show the student how to lengthen and bring freedom to the body. The author notes that the National Health Service uses the technique and that many physicians refer patients to Alexander Technique teachers. A case for nurses, midwives, and health visitors to learn the technique's benefits is made.

Valentine, Elisabeth R., et al. "The Effect of Lessons in the Alexander Technique on Music Performance in High and Low Stress Situations." *Psychology of Music* **23, no. 2 (1995): 129–41.**
This article describes a scientific study of the application of the Alexander Technique in musical performance lessons. Twenty-five students with various instruments, including voice, cello, piano, organ, flute, oboe, clarinet, and trombone, were divided into an experimental and control group on a random basis. Experimental measurements were applied and recorded on four separate occasions, two at low-stress points (in class prior to treatment and in class after treatment) and two at high-stress points (audition and recital) for students in both groups. The experimental group received fifteen lessons in the Alexander Technique, while the control, though aware of the design and treatment, did not receive any technique instruction. The subjects completed the Eysneck Personality Inventory and the Performance Anxiety Inventory. They also rated their interest in having Alexander Technique lessons. At each of the stress points, all subjects were measured for height and peak flow (peak expiratory flow, a measure of the pressure exerted in forced expiration) because of claims that the Alexander Technique increases the realization of potential height and improves breath control. Subjects' heart rates were also gauged as a measure of arousal under stress. Subjects also self-reported their mood, using the Full Nowlis Mood Adjective checklist. The study found that the main hypothesis, that the Alexander Technique would increase height or peak flow or modulate the increase in mean heart rate under stress, was not proven and no effects were found to be statistically significant. However, the experimental group did show improvement from preclass to postclass relative to control on overall technical quality.

5

Electronic Resources on the Alexander Technique

Alexander Technique, at www.life.uiuc.edu/jeff/alextech.html.
This page acts as a wonderful springboard for those interested in learning more about the Alexander Technique. The site contains links to descriptions of the technique from the American Society for the Alexander Technique and Alexander Technique International, as well as several informative links to the Alexander Technique Center of Washington, D.C. There are also many links to various professional organizations around the world, as well as links to journal and printing press sources that focus on the technique.

Alexander Technique Center, at www.alexandercenter.com/.
This site has a wealth of information regarding the technique, with clear links to information on the history of the technique, the benefits of learning it, teacher training programs, lessons and workshops, literature and materials, and book reviews. There is even a specific link for musicians, which breaks up several sections of links to information and literature into categories for singers, string players, and woodwind players. This subsection also includes links to articles and literature specifically for musicians.

Alexander Technique International, at www.ati-net.com/.
This site is a very good resource for those who wish to stay informed with up-to-date information on what is going on in the world of Alexander Technique (AT). It is open to teachers and nonteachers alike. The only requirements are that one be certified in AT and pay membership dues. The website contains links to articles, information on workshops and how to locate teachers worldwide, links to published resources, and the *Journal of Alexander Technique International*, "Ex-Change."

Alexander Technique in the UK, www.stat.org.uk/.

This site is the official website of the Society of Teachers of the Alexander Technique (STAT), the British Alexander Technique organization. The website acts as the informational contact for STAT and its activities. The front page includes numerous links that connect to descriptions of various principles and aspects of the Alexander Technique, with navigation on the left-hand side, including the purpose of the technique, what occurs in a typical lesson, advice on finding a teacher, a history of the origins and development of the technique, an FAQ link, a webliography, and a description of STAT as an organization.

American Center for the Alexander Technique, at www.acatnyc.org/.

Founded in New York City in 1964, the American Center for the Alexander Technique has taken a leading role in the development of the Alexander Technique in the United States, not only through its Teacher Certification Program, but also through its thirty years of service to the public as an information, resource, and referral center, and also through its ongoing commitment to the standards and ideals of the Alexander Technique. The Teacher Certification Program of the American Center is licensed by the New York State Bureau of Proprietary Schools and is also an approved training course of the American Society for the Alexander Technique (AmSAT). This site is primarily geared toward those interested in attending this institution to attain certification, though it does contain information regarding the history and basic concepts behind the technique. Also contained are links to the two leading American Alexander websites.

Rickover, Robert. "Alexander Technique Teacher Training: A Comprehensive Guide," at http://thealexandertechnique.net/.

The purpose of this site is to provide information for those seeking training in the Alexander Technique. It is run by a teacher who started his training in the 1970s and whose intent is to lessen the difficulty of getting started for those who would like to begin their training. The site provides clear links to (1) Locate Alexander Technique Teacher Training Courses, (2) Information and Advice about the Training Process, (3) Resources for Alexander Technique Teachers and Students, (4) General Information about the Alexander Technique, and (5) A Note to Alexander Technique Teachers and Training Course Directors.

Rickover, Robert, and Anne Rickover. "Complete Guide to the Alexander Technique," at www.alexandertechnique.com/.

This site is written and maintained by Robert and Anne Rickover, well-known Alexander Technique teachers, who are frequent contributors to *Direction*, the prime journal on the Alexander Technique. They ask the viewers of the site four questions about their body health, including whether or not they suffer from back pain, repetitive motion injuries, discomfort when sitting, and on occupations related to use of the Alexander Technique. The site provides numerous links to articles that explain principles and issues directly related to the technique, including (1) an explanation of the Alexander Technique, (2) how to find a teacher or course, (3) an explanation of typical class events, (4) the musician and the Alexander Technique, (5) medical and scientific research on the technique and print, video, and journal resources, (6) an Alexander Technique online bookstore, (7) interactive resources available on the Web, (8) numerous essays on the principles of the technique, and (9) a biography of F. M. Alexander. They also provide links to four related sites: (1) ergonomics, (2) physical therapy and the Alexander Technique, (3) a comprehensive guide to Alexander Technique Teacher Training, and (4) Pilates and the Alexander Technique.

Westminster Alexander Centre, at www.alextech.demon.co.uk/.
This site is the homepage for an Alexander Technique school in Central London. It provides links to information regarding the basic tenets for the technique, as well as information on contacting the teachers. Of special importance are the links to articles the teachers have written, which give a more in-depth explanation of the technique and its necessity, especially to musicians (www.alextech. demon.co.uk/wac202.htm).

6

Journals on the Alexander Technique and Body-Work Subjects

There are very few journals and serial publications dedicated exclusively to the Alexander Technique. The best journal is *Direction*, published in Australia by Direction Journal. This title is published twice per year, beginning in 1988, and its contents are entirely concerned with topics on the Alexander Technique. The second most important journal is the *Alexander Journal*, the official publication of STAT: the Society of Teachers of the Alexander Technique, the British Alexander Technique society. There are also two important newsletters from the largest of the Alexander Technique societies in the United States: (1) *In the Moment* (formerly *AuSTAT News*), the newsletter of the Australian Society of Teachers of the Alexander Technique and (2) *AMSAT News*, the newsletter of the American Society for the Alexander Technique.

This chapter provides a list of the articles in each issue of *Direction*, and where the article or abstract could be examined, a brief synopsis of the article is provided. In addition to the articles in *Direction*, the publishing information for several Alexander Technique and body-work journals are provided. The body-work journals have been included as these titles occasionally discuss the Alexander Technique and its related principles. Also included are the contents of each of the issues of the *Alexander Review*.

DIRECTION, PUBLISHED BY PAUL COOK AND DIRECTION JOURNAL. ISSN: 1039-3145.

Vol. 1, No. 1, Premier Issue

Auburn, P. "Feldenkrais and Alexander"
Kaufman, S. "A Personal Comparison"

Leeper, A. "The Leeper Report"
McLeod, R. "Australia since "F.M."
McLeod, R. "The Critical Moment"

Vol. 1, No. 2, Marjorie Barstow Issue

Alexander, F. M. "The Prevention and Cure of Consumption." Previously published, Alexander was known as " Breathing Man" because he espoused "the perfect respiratory treatment."

Brenner, W. "Practical Marj." Interview of Marjory Barlow at age seventy-nine.

Chance, J. "A Teacher's Perspective of Feelings." Chance, the journal's editor,
describes the influence of Barstow in his teachings.

Chance, V., and M. Llewyllen. "Marj in Australia: Pictures and Aphorisms."
Barstow notes, "Learn to laugh at yourselves: you always move better with a smile."

Clark, Jean. "Words as Communication." The importance of words in teaching the
technique.

Stenning, M. "Peace and the Alexander Technique." The author cautions about
seeking to control outer things.

Vol. 1, No. 3, Dart Issue

Alexander, F. M. "New Method of Vocal Respiratory Re-education." Alexander's
second paper in a series of three articles on respiration (the first available in vol.
1, no. 2, and the third in vol. 1, no. 4).

Hough, A. "Voice and the Alexander Technique." Based on Husler's work, he argues
that evolutionary origins of singing challenge conventional Alexander thinking.

Lord, K. J. "Disunity in the United States." An examination of the organizational
split between two main Alexander organizations in the United States.

Murray, A. "The Dart Procedures." A practical guide to Raymond Dart's work, including illustrations.

Nicolson, A., R. Simmons, and C. Raff. "Teaching the Procedures." The Dart procedures are explained for use on oneself as well as others.

Raff, C. "A Lengthening Tune in Adelaide." Report of an experimental project
with musicians at the University of Adelaide.

Tobias, P. "Tribute to Raymond Dart." Tobias pays tribute to Dart. Tobias was
Dart's successor at Witwatersrand University.

Wheelhouse, F. "Dart and Alexander." A biographical review of Dart's lifelong
interest in poise.

Vol. 1, No. 4, Walter Carrington Issue

Alexander, F. M. "Respiratory Re-education"
Carrington, W. "The Australian Influence"
Garlick, D. "Brighton Lectures, Part 1"
Holland, M. "Walter Carrington, a Portrait"
Mixan, L. and Burton, F. "Sensory Perception"
Nicholls, L. "Interview: Dilys Carrington"
———. "Interview: Walter Carrington"
———. "Walter's Talk"

Vol. 1, No. 5, Brighton Congress

Ballard, K. "Postural Reflexes." The author discusses postural reflexes of the feet within the context of the Alexander Technique.

Caplan, D. "Back Pain and How to Cope." The author discusses back pain and its relief from a physical therapy perspective and the Alexander Technique.

Macdonald, G. "We Go Forward and Up." A discussion of the whispered "ah" from one of the most renown Alexander Technique authors.

Price-Williams, D. "Loss of Innocence." The use and influence of language in movement reeducation. The author questions the effects of communication and teaching.

Rathbone, M. "An Early History of Alexander." A biographical discussion of F. M. Alexander's family roots.

Trevelyan, G. "Act. Don't React." Trevelyan describes the Alexander Technique in his own unique way, including humor and poetry.

Vol. 1, No. 6, Kids and Pregnancy

Ackers, K. "Fortune Cookie"
Fischer, J. "F. M. Alexander and Evolution"
Garlick, D. "The Sub-Cortical Centres"
Liedloff, J. "The Continuum Concept"
Machover, I. "The Alexander Way to Eutokia"
Madden, C. "A Perspective to Parenting"
Scott, S. "A Positive Approach to Children"
Sokolsky, M. "Pregnancy and the AT"
Tobias, P. "Posture and Locomotion"

Vol. 1, No. 7, Feldenkrais and Alexander Issue

Fischer, J. "F. M. Alexander and Evolution." Jean Fischer writes that bemusement may give way to disgust when reading the seriously proposed racist aspect of Alexander's evolutionary theories.

Hall, D. "Awareness through Movement." ATM is the Feldenkrais version of exercise but is nothing you ever imagined: you lie on the floor, roll around, listen to your body, and experiment with movement.

——. "The Pursuit of Poise." David Hall, a practitioner of both methods, offers thought-provoking ideas on professional chauvinism, compulsive behavior, and pain while exploring each technique.

——. "What Is the Feldenkrais Method?" Hall interviews a leading Feldenkrais practitioner Mark Reese, who asks obvious questions and explores its relationship to Alexander's work.

Johnson-Chase, M. "Musings on the Methods." Michael Johnson-Chase postulates on the two methods: do they show two types of scientific thinking: divergent and convergent creativity?

Tobias, P. "Man the Tottering Biped: Anatomy of Posture in Higher Primates." The sweeping evolutionary adaptations for bipedalism are reviewed in the second of Professor Phillip Tobias's five-part series.

Vol. 1, No. 8, Music and Musicians Issue

Benedetti, E. "Playing in a Symphony." The author describes her experience learning the Alexander Technique with the guidance of Leonard Bernstein while a member of the New York Philharmonic.

Ben-Or, N. "Conceptions and Misconceptions." A discussion of common myths and misconceptions of the Alexander Technique in concert piano instruction.

Mackie, V. "Butterfly Soup." Mackie, a student of Pablo Casals, describes how she learned to create her musical output by learning to stay in the moment and how Casals's teaching on this related to her experiences with the Alexander Technique.

Mathews, T. "Blessed Helicity." The author describes Raymond Dart's principles of anatomy, especially the double-helical structure of our musculature, or the spirals that integrate our movement system.

McGee, M. "How to Play Beethoven." A discussion of learning to play Beethoven by applying the Alexander Technique.

Rickover, R. "Self Help Alexander." A discussion of learning the Alexander Technique alone.

Tobias, P. "Man the Tottering Biped: Part III—What the Fossils Tell Us." An examination of how the fossil record is used to understand the evolutionary development of bipedalism.

Vol. 1, No. 9, Emotions Issue

Chance, J. "The Anatomy of Addiction." A discussion of alcoholism and how the Alexander Technique helped with this malady.

Crow, A. "Dreambody and Alexander Work." This article examines the emotions and whether or not Alexander Technique principles create a limitation in dealing with mood.

Johnson-Chase, M. "Do We Cry Because We Grieve, or Do We Grieve Because We Cry?" The author discusses the role of emotions in creating a character in acting and theater settings, utilizing his experiences with the Alexander and Feldenkrais techniques.

Morris, W. C. "Hazards and Hope." An Alexander teacher describes how her exploration of the technique helped her cope with an abusive past.

Rubenfeld, I. "Emotions: The Unacknowledged Partner." The author, a world-renown Alexander Technique expert, describes her development of "Synergy," emotional body work.

Tobias, P. "Man the Tottering Biped: Part IV—Uprightness, Gravity, and Balance." Part 4 of the author's series on how the fossil record is used to understand the evolutionary development of bipedalism.

Vol. 1, No. 10, Dance and Movement Issue

Arnold, M. "False Self." A discussion and review of two articles on emotion that appeared in *Direction* 1, no. 9.

Bondy, P. "The Space Between: Stimulus and Response." The author describes her experiences as a student and teacher of the Alexander Technique.

Crow, A. "Authentic Movement." Crow discusses tension patterns and the importance of recognizing them.

Diamond, J. "The Actor and the Neutral State." The acting concept of a "neutral state" is examined.

Garren, E. "Sometime Wrestling . . . Always Dancing." A personal account of the author's professional and personal struggles, with emphasis on a dance career.

Karczag, E. "As Yet Untitled." The author, a renowned leader in experimental dance and an Alexander teacher, describes her views of the technique as it applies to dance.

Murrow, L. "Dance Therapy." The author promotes psychotherapeutic movement to improve physical and emotional integration.

Paludan, M. "Marjorie Barstow Interviewed by Marsha Paludan." Barstow describes her experiences with dance within the context of Alexander Technique lessons, especially from F. M. Alexander.

Tobias, P. "Man the Tottering Biped: Part V—The Skilled Use of the Body." Part 5 of the author's series on how the fossil record is used to understand the evolutionary development of bipedalism.

Vol. 2, No. 1, Equitation Issue

Clark, J. "Are You Sitting Comfortably?"
Faraldi, L. "Dressage Links"
Garlick, D. "Lengthening"
Harris, C. "Three Functional Centres"
Long, M. "Alexander Leeper"
Pevsner, D. "A Lesson in Horsemanship"
Roberts, T. "Balance and Gravity"
Swift, S. "Personal History"
Tobias, P. "Skilled Use of Body"
Tottle, S. "Working with Mr. Spooks"
Weis, R. "What's It All About?"

Vol. 2, No. 2, The Barlows Issue

Battye, A. "Doctor Barlow." Battye survived a car accident with the aid of Alexander Technique instruction from Dr. Barlow.

Brockbank, N. "Conscious Control." The author argues that teachers are often unaware of the true nature of "conscious control."

Garlick, D. "Semi-Supine." Garlick, best known for his review of research on the Alexander Technique, describes the benefits from health of the spinal vertebrae to decreases in heart rate and blood pressure.

Grey, J. "We Might Be Able to Help." Grey, a well-known actor, recounts his instruction on the technique from Marjory Barlow.

Oxford, F. "Marjory Barlow Interviewed." An interview with Marjory Barlow, including numerous anecdotes about F. M. Alexander.

Tobias, P. "Man the Tottering Biped: Part VI—The Role of the Nervous System." The final installment of the author's series on how the fossil record is used to understand the evolutionary development of bipedalism.

Walker, E. "Fifty-five Years On." Walker describes her travels to South Africa, meeting Nelson Mandela, and her experiences learning the Alexander Technique.

Vol. 2, No. 3, Voice Issue

Arcava, B. "Training the Singing Voice." The author, an opera singer and Alexander Technique teacher, examines the work of Manuel Garcia.

Caine, A. "What's the Matter? Lost Your Tongue?" Caine argues that Alexander lessons will not improve the voice without improving habits of the tongue.

Champ, J. "Breathe Easy, Breathe Low." Champ describes ways of improving breathing with the Alexander Technique as well as lessons from her own voice training.

Dennis, R. "Breathe from Your Diaphragm and Other Myths." An iconoclastic view of voice training, exposing some of the myths of the profession.

Hjortshoj, K. "Language and Movement." The author questions the effects of his own Alexander training and considers whether his voice difficulties weren't exacerbated by this instruction.

Joudry, R. "The Use of the Ear." An account of Alfred Tomatis, who posited new ideas about the ear's function and of reeducating the use of listening through the Alexander Technique.

McCallion, M. "Voice Lost." The author critiques the poor instruction of Alexander Technique teachers on the voice and argues that most Alexander teaching does not improve the voice.

Vol. 2, No. 4, Sexuality Issue

Barstow, M. "Aphorisms of Marjorie Barstow." A collection of comments and sayings from Marjorie Barstow.

Diamond, J. "Sex and Love Addicts." The author explores her own path of inhibition and of addiction through lessons learned as an Alexander Technique student and teacher.

Flechas, A. "Sex Habits and How to Break Them." A discourse challenging the claim that the Alexander Technique can rehabilitate sex offenders.

Hanefeld, N. "We Are Sexless, Not!" The author argues that sexuality and gender play a role in client relations during instruction as well as instruction itself.

Hannan, K. "There's More between the Hips Than Meets the Hands." A personal account of a bisexual lesbian and her encounters with more conservative individuals in Alexander Technique circles.

Heenan, C. "Sexuality? Whose?" An account of bias against gays and lesbians by STAT, the Society of Teachers of the Alexander Technique.

McDowell, J., and W. Bonington. "Ethical Issues of Sexual Contact." An interview with Mary Cox on the issues teachers and therapists face with developing friendships with clients.

Rahtz, G. "Boys on Bike." The author discusses teacher/therapist relations with clients, especially physical attraction concerns.

Stallibrass, C. "A Survey of Sex." A report of a study of attitudes of sexuality and practices after receiving Alexander Technique training.

Staring, J. "F. M. Alexander and Samuel Butler." Staring examines the charge that F. M. Alexander was a racist and examines his relationship with Samuel Butler, who greatly influenced Alexander on his views about race.

Vol. 2, No. 5, Macdonald and the Israelis Issue

Borst, C. "Scott's Teaching Aphorisms." The author recounts his training by Scott.

Diamond, J. "The Israeli Director." Diamond describes the teaching styles of five Israeli Alexander Technique teachers.

Kaminitz, S. "Mr. Macdonald (1910–1991)." The author recounts her training experiences under the tutelage of Patrick Macdonald.

———. "On Feet Wide Apart." Kaminitz offers her insight into Macdonald's style of teaching that focuses on sitting and standing with legs placed wide apart.

Mausner, R., and J. Cohen. "Effects of Childhood Trauma." This article examines whether the Alexander Technique training can trigger forgotten traumatic experiences.

Morton, W. "Mr. Scott (1918–1978)." Morton began his experiences with the Alexander Technique as an assistant to Patrick Macdonald, and he tells his story about these experiences.

Webster, M. "A Tale of Two Trainings." Webster trained under Macdonald and then Scott. He describes and compares his experiences.

Vol. 2, No. 6, Spirituality Issue

Polatin, B. "The Place We Never Leave." Polatin analyzes spiritual practice and Alexander practice.

Roberts, T. D. M. "Reflexes, Habits, and Skills." Roberts examines the meaning of terms he has often found applied in an incorrect way.

Rumme, D. "Stepping off a 100-Foot Pole—Beyond the Limits of Reason and Faith." Rumme, a monk, explores the spiritual side of the Alexander Technique, including issues of religion and science.

Walshe, R. D. "Every Moment Alexander." The author explains what links John Dewey, Krishnamurti, Lao Tzu, Gurdjieff, Rudolf Steiner, F. M. Alexander, A. E. Housman, and humanistic psychology.

Vol. 2, No. 7, Vision Issue

Carrington, W., with B. Cavadias and M. Fern. "The Use of the Eye." Carrington describes the primary importance of the eye with Bridgette Cavadias and Marjorie Fern.

Cavadias, B. "William Horatio's Brainwave." The author discusses Bates's advocacy of vision as "a bunch of end-gaining exercises."

Freeman, B. "The How and Why of the Eye." The author argues that the eye as an organ "designed for seeing" is an inappropriate concept.

Gauld, L. "Perfect Grace." Gauld describes Aldous Huxley's work with Alexander and Bates to improve his vision and health.

Grunwald, P. "The Eye-Body Reflex Patterns." Grunwald maps links between the eye and the body from his own discovery process of shortening and narrowing his cornea.

Pollock, C. "Have a Ball." Pollock describes how a new stimulus freshens the response and thinking in an Alexander Technique lesson.

Vol. 2, No. 8, Multiculturalism

Alexander, R. "Black and White." Riki recounts the incident whereby some NA-STAT (now AmSTAT) members attempted to denounce some passages in Alexander's *Man's Supreme Inheritance* as racist and insensitive to the races.

Batson, G. "Sticking to Principle—Teaching Alexander in Ecuador." Batson describes the cultural challenges of teaching the Alexander Technique in Ecuador.

Freeman, M. F. "Moving beyond Words: Working with People Who "Listen" by Watching." Freeman describes how sign language is used in Alexander Technique teaching.

Gilmore, R. "Crossing Hemispheres—Forward and Up with the Rising Sun." Gilmore was the director of KAPPA, a four-year training program for teachers of the Alexander work in Japan. In this article, she describes the cultural challenges of teaching the technique to the Japanese.

Rossi, R. L., and C. Madden. "Zweimal Frühstuck Bitte." Rossi and Madden provide a comparative view of multicultural teaching in Europe. Rossi questions the need for teaching in English.

Sheldon, F. "Living in the Present." An interview with Hella Linkmeyer on her work with African bushmen, where she visited the !Kung (click your tongue) bushmen of the Kalahari Desert in Namibia.

Thompson, T. "An Alexander Way of Life." A discussion of Alexander Technique as a way of life in a multicultural world.

Waldman, M. "A Classical Use of the Front Hand." Waldman describes his analysis of Patrick Macdonald's use of his front hand while teaching. A photoset of this hand use is included.

Vol. 2, No. 9, Spirituality II Issue

Alexander, W. "A Spiritual Path." Alexander examines the similarities and differences of the Alexander Technique and "A Course in Miracles" and concludes that it is crucial to define "mind." He argues that these two programs seem to conflict with each other.

Cash, D. "The Path Is Always Present." A discourse of the "promise of tshuvah" and the Alexander Technique, learning to change mind and body.

Gorman, D. "The Rounder We Go, the Samer We Get [part one]." This two-part series is based on a lecture given at the Centre for Training and discusses the nature of circular habits and how to escape them.

Hadar-Borthwick, M. "Working with Aliens." A personal account of the author working with a client with a mixture of therapy, spirituality, and the Alexander Technique.

Martin, H. "Syncronising Body and Mind." The author examines the similarities and differences of the Alexander Technique and Buddhist meditation, two practices that lead the mind and body into direct relationship.

Protzel, M. "A Kinaesthetic Venture." Protzel recounts his experiences discovering the life-changing value of the Alexander Technique.

Vol. 2, No. 10, The Future Issue

Bruce, L. "Our Brains Beguiled"
Cacciatore, T. "Science and Alexander"
Engel, F. "On General Principle"
Fitzgerald, T. "Teacher Education: Part 1"
Gorman, D. "The Rounder We Go, Part 1"
Kettrick, C. "Six Master Teachers Interviewed"

Vol. 3, No. 1, Yoga Issue

Chapman, K. "Off the Table: An Alexander Teacher on the Mat." Chapman describes Western yoga as end-gaining at its worst, from her experiences as a yoga instructor for more than thirty years and an Alexander teacher for the past twenty years.

Charlson, L. "Interview: Michael Frederick and Sigrid Wagner." Frederick, an Alexander Technique teacher, and Wagner, a yoga instructor, compare and contrast the two techniques in this interview.

Fawlkner, S. "Of One Mind: Alexander and Ashtanga." Fawlkner finds that the philosophical basis for Alexander Technique and yoga are the same, except for one aspect, which he discusses.

Fitzgerald, T. "Alexander Teacher Education [part two]." Fitzgerald poses questions and answer concerning accreditation, competency-based assessment, and professional profiles for Alexander Technique instruction.

Hook, D. "Yoking the East and West." Melding Eastern approaches to yoga with Western practice, Hook describes how to bring yoga into daily life activities.

Thompson, K. "Discovering Yoga." Thompson describes the growth of interest in yoga and suggests ways to begin thinking how to approach it as a practice.

Waldman, M. "Formulation of an Alexander Lesson, Part 1." Waldman, a practicing naturopath and osteopath, suggests approaches to beginning a training session with a new pupil.

Vol. 3, No. 2, Performance Issue

Laurie, S. "Working with Actors." The author describes her work with actors at the Royal Shakespeare Company and the Royal National Theatre.

Madden, C. "Integrated Actor Training." A description of the University of Washington's actor training program and the integration of the Alexander Technique in the program's instruction.

Pollock, C. "Aikido: Exploring the Space of Inhibition." Pollock describes the lessons from combining an understanding of Aikido and the Alexander Technique.

Rodrigue, J. "A Coach for All Seasons." An interview with Kelly McEvenue on her work at the Straford Repertory Theatre in Canada and her instruction on the Alexander Technique.

———. "The Naked Truth: Ann Stocking: A Case History." A case study of a disabled actress and her acting training, aided by the principles of the Alexander Technique.

Sly, M. "Professionalism: Compromising Principles." The author reviews the professional literature on certification and accreditation efforts of the Alexander Technique and the debate on this subject.

Waldman, M. "An Alexander Lesson, Part II." Through walking, table turns, the whispered "ah," and rhythm, the diversity of an Alexander lesson is described.

Wolf, J. "The Breathing Costume." A unique group teaching method at Yale University is described that aids actors and their breathing.

Vol. 3, No. 3, Business and Marketing Issue

Vol. 3, No. 4, Paradigms of Self Issue

THE ALEXANDER JOURNAL (CONTENTS PAGES OF EACH ISSUE)

Issue 21 (March 2006)

Contents: "Accompanying Alexander" by Alex Farkas, "Alexander in Professional Dance" by Michael Schumacher, "First of the Second Generation" by Joyce Bird, "Working with Actors 2" by Lee Warren, "Inhibition" anthologized by Jean Fischer with an introduction by Francesca Greenoak, "Preliminary Research into Head and Shoulder Balance in Dancers" by Sarah Irvine, "Lost in Translation" by Harriet Anderson, "The Impact of Psychotherapy and Counselling on the Alexander Technique" by Brigitta Mowat, "Effects of the Alexander Technique on Muscle Activation" by Elyse Shafarman.

Issue 20 (Summer 2003)

Contents: "Candles and Onions: Layers of Learning" by Carolyn Nicholls, "Working with Groups" by Lee Warren, "The Alexander Technique and Traumatic Injury" by Kathryn Zimmerman, "An Appreciation of Marjory Barlow's Examined Life" by Mike Cross, "Skiing and the Alexander Technique" by Maggie Lamb, "Primary Control" collated by Jean Fischer with an introduction by Francesca Greenoak, "Lying Semi-supine" by Francesca Greenoak, "Making Connections" by Malcolm Williamson.

Issue 19 (Spring 2003)

Contents: "Making the Link" by John Hunter, "The Application of the Alexander Technique to Piano Teaching" by Rudolf Kratzert, "Thoughts on Musicians and the Alexander Technique" by Elizabeth Langford, "Primum Mobile" poem by Bobbie Gallagher, "Helena's First Lessons" by Carolyn Nicholls, "Dance and the Alexander Technique" by Rachel Rist, "How the Use of the Self Triumphed over Dependence on a Machine" by Madeleine Samuelson-White, "The Alexander Technique and Traumatic Injury" by Kathryn Zimmerman.

Issue 18 (Summer 2002)

Contents: "The Adventures of Leg and His Companion Voice" by Michael Mc-Callion, "The Primary Matter in Buddhism and the Alexander Technique" by

Mike Cross, "Textural Note: Inhibition" by Ray Evans, "The Alexander Technique and Riding" by Lesley Finn-Kelcey, "Alexander and the Alexander Technique: Reminiscences" by V. Jagannathan, "Thy Fingers Walk with Gentle Gait: Reading the Sonnet" by Lawrence Bruce, "Out of the Chair: An Alexander Teacher on the Run" by Malcolm Balk, "Down Is a Four-Letter Word: Distillations from Workshops" by Nelly Ben-Or.

Issue 17 (Summer 2001)

Contents: "Uncharted Waters: The Alexander Technique and Swimming" by Steven Shaw, "Invisible Women" by Terry Fitzgerald, "Robert Thayer's Work on Mood and Arousal in the Context of the Alexander Technique" by Richard Casebow, "Textural Note" by Jean-Do Masoero and Francesca Greenoak, "The Use of the Chair" by Christl Moffat, "Feet Up" by students and teachers at the Alexander Re-education Centre, "Posture Tension and Technique" by Niso Ticciati.

Issue 16 (1999)

Contents: "F. M. Alexander's Training Course" by Tony Spawforth, "The Eyes and the Primary Control" by Kathleen Ballard, "Inhibition in the Picture Gallery" by Kerry Downes, "The Searchlight of Attention" by Kevan Martin, "Handwriting" by Jonathan Drake, "Recollections by a Pupil of Alexander's" by Cliff Lewis, "A Pupil's Notebook" by Penny Lyons and Alex Down.

Issue 15 (1997)

Contents: "Our Journey to South Africa" by Elisabeth Walker, "The Essence of F. M.'s Teaching" by Marjory Barlow, "Nice Voice, Pity about the Words" by Alexander Farkas, "Alexander and Montessori" by Nicola Hanefeld.

Issue 14 (1995)

Contents: "F. M. Alexander as I Knew Him" by Walter Carrington, "Alexander's Discoveries and What We Have Made of Them" by Adam Nott, "The Use of the Self" by Pedro de Alcantara, "Odent in the Light of the Alexander Technique" by Masoumeh Atabaki and Ilana Machover, "Working with a Cancer Support Group" by Penny Ingham, "A Radical View of Sitting" by Nicholas Brockbank, and "Movement versus Rest" by Marianne Marshall.

Issue 13 (1993)

Contents: "Alexander's way" by Erika Whittaker, "Aesthetic Re-education" by Alexander Farkas, "'This Alarming Cult'" by "Screwtape," "To a Child at the Piano" poem by Alastair Reid, "The True Wholeness" by Sir George Trevelyan.

Issue 12 (1992)

Contents: "A Personal View of the Alexander Technique" by Misha Magidov, "A Personal View of the Alexander Technique" by Sir George Trevelyan, "The Alexander Technique in the Kindergarten" by Laura Harwood, "'Alexander's gloom': A Case History" by Linda Gillard.

Issue 11 (1991)

Contents: "Why I Took Up Alexander's Work" by Sir George Trevelyan, "A Pianist's Adventure with the Alexander Technique" by Nelly Ben-Or, "What Is Inhibition" by Nicholas Brockbank, "Poem: The Alexander Technique" by Jean de Heger, "The Alexander Technique and Dance" by Phyllis G. Richmond, "Don't Do It but Do the Don't" by Jean M. O. Fischer, "A Way to Spontaneous Living" by Ruth Borchard.

Issue 10 (1989)

Contents: "Finding Meaning in One's Work" by Shmuel Nelken, "On Categorising the Alexander Technique" by Walter Carrington, "Learning to Apply the Technique" by Nicholas Brockbank, "Greater Awareness in Pregnancy" by Nicola Hanefeld, "The Use and Abuse of Anatomy" by Joel Carbonel, "What We Can Expect from 1992" by Stephen Jupp, "Fixed Ideas about Being Free" by Beauchamp Bagenal.

Issue 9 (1988)

Contents: "Eileen French: An Appreciation" by Nina E. C. Coltart, "On Giving Directions, Doing, and Non-doing" by Patrick Macdonald, "What F. M. Alexander Said about Right and Wrong," "Eavesdropping" by Jean Clark, "Stanislavsky and the Alexander Technique" by Nicolette Lee, "The Alexander Technique and Psychotherapy" by John Naylor, "Man's Presumptuous Brain" by Ruth Borchard.

Issue 8 (1978)

Contents: "Some Reflections on F. M. Alexander" by M. E. Coaker, "A Pianist's Thoughts on the Alexander Technique" by Nelly Ben-Or, "Coming to Know" by Dr. Philida Salmon, "Talking about the Technique" by Jean Clark, "The Philosopher's Stone" by James Harvey Robinson, "The Value of Misuse" by Dorothea Wallis, "Physiological Gradients" by A. Rugg-Gunn.

Issue 7 (1972)

Contents: Extracts from Alexander's writings: "Conscious Guidance and Control," "Use and Change," "Use and Health," "Terms Used in the Technique," "Standing, Walking, and Sitting," and "Teaching Aphorism."

Issue 6 (1968)

Contents: "Tributes to Miss Tasker," "An Unrecognised Need in Education" by Irene Tasker, "The Attainment of Poise" by Raymond Dart, "The South African Legal Action" by Dr. Wilfred Barlow, "Recording a Miracle" by Louise Morgan, "The Deeper Significance of Posture and Movement" by Dr. Grahame Fagg.

Issue 5 (1966)

Contents: "Alexander's Empiricism" by Walter Carrington, "Mr. Alexander's Use of Scientific Method" by A. R. Heath, "Technique in Industry" by Robert Best, "The First Twelve Lessons" by anonymous, "Relaxation of Muscle Tension" by Dr. D. R. Price-Williams.

Issue 4 (1965)

Contents: "Foreword" by F. Matthias Alexander, "Instinct and Functioning in Health and Disease" by Peter Macdonald, "The F. Matthias Alexander Technique and Its Relation to Education" by I. G. Griffith, "End-gaining and Means-Whereby" by Aldous Huxley, "F. Matthias Alexander and the Problem of Animal Behaviour" by A. Rugg-Gunn, "The Work of F. M. Alexander and the Medical White Paper" by D. S. Radcliffe Drew, "Knowing How to Stop" by Wilfred Barlow, "The F. Matthias Alexander Technique" by Frank Pierce Jones.

Issue 3 (1964)

Contents: "Alexander's View of Psycho-analysis" by Marjory Barlow, "Jung and Alexander: The Common Ground" by Nina Meyer, "The Process of Growth" by Robin Skynner, "Preoccupation with the Disconnected" by John Dewey, "Where Golfers Go Wrong" by Sir Ernest Holderness, "The Indirect Competition to Singing" by Joyce Warrack, Obituary: Aldous Huxley, "Alexander's Meeting with Coghill" by Edward H. Owen.

Issue 2 (1963)

Contents: "The Technique and Back Disorders" by Eric de Peyer, "Alexander and the Mastery of Habit" by Edward H. Owen, "What F. M. Alexander Said about Habit and Change," "The Barrier of Habit" by John Dewey, "Some Varieties of Mis-use" by Wilfred Barlow, "Education without 'End-gaining'" by Irene Tasker.

Issue 1 (1962)

Contents: "Tribute to a 'Great Teacher'" by Sir Stafford Cripps, "Psycho-physical Integrity" by Patrick J. Macdonald, "The Technique in Drama: Tension and the

Actor" by Joyce Wodeman, "Right and Wrong: Sayings of F. M. Alexander," "A Higher Education" by Paul Work, "The Physical Foundations of Spiritual Growth" by Aldous Huxley, "A Ring at the Door" by Dorothea Wallis.

ALEXANDER TECHNIQUE NEWSLETTERS OF IMPORTANCE

The ACAT Newsletter
AMSTAT News

7

Audiovisual Materials

Audiovisual materials provide a visual means for learning the technique. The materials included in this chapter constitute the titles that can be accessed from a library, as indexed in the online database, WorldCat, which includes a listing of libraries that own these titles in their collections. These items are by no means all the available audiovisual materials. Most Alexander Technique associations and many Alexander Technique training schools and teachers have audiovisual materials that are useful for learning the technique. It is best to search the Web pages of the primary Alexander Technique associations to locate other materials.

Alexander, F. Matthias, and John A. Baron. *Use of the Self.* Audio cassette tapes. Tiburon, Calif.: Big Sur Tapes, 1996.

American Choral Directors' Association. *Alexander Technique.* Audio cassette tapes. Clarence, N.Y.: Mark Custom Recording, 1990.

Beaton, Brian, Celia Tate, and Serene Lim. *The Nature of Healing, Vol. 1.* DVD. Huntingdon, UK: Quantum Leap, 1996.
The *Nature of Healing* looks at "alternative" medical treatments from a range of cultures including China, India, Japan, and Sweden—treatments that are gaining acceptance among orthodox practitioners and their patients. Three subjects are covered in this program: acupuncture, meditation, and movement.

Caplan, Deborah. *The Alexander Technique: Solutions for Back Trouble.* VHS. New York: Wellspring Media, 1998.
Offers specific and practical guidance in how to help you keep your back healthy and free from pain by using the Alexander Technique.

Chance, Jeremy. *Principles of the Alexander Technique.* Audio cassette tape. London: Thorsons Audio, 1999.

———. *Thorsons Principles of Alexander Technique.* Audio cassette tape. London: Thorsons Audio, 1999.

Conable, Barbara, William Conable, and Susan Stratton. *How to Learn the Alexander Technique: A Manual for Students.* Audio cassette tape. Columbus, Ohio: Andover Press, 1997.

Craig, Valda, Louise Willis, and Tony Geeves. *Smart Dance.* VHS. Walsh Bay, Australia: Ausdance, 1993.
Advice for dancers on achieving maximal performance and lengthening careers through good technique and training, nutrition, and injury prevention.

Dowling, Niamh. *Alexander Technique into Performance.* VHS. Exeter, UK: Arts Documentation Unit, 1999.
Niamh Dowling trained as a teacher of the Alexander Technique and with Monika Pagneux in Paris. This video is a record of a workshop she gave to a group of performers at the London Studio Centre. The workshop was based on the principles of the Alexander Technique both as a preparation for work and as a technical basis from which to release performance.

Duncan, Lindsay. Commentary. *The Art of Swimming: The Shaw Method.* VHS. London: Odyssey Video, 1998.
The Art of Swimming is the first film to present the Shaw Method of Swimming, which integrates swimming with the Alexander Technique. It highlights the benefit of swimming as the ideal remedy for stress.

Galardi, Toni, Greg Holdaway, Petra Schaefer, and Claudio Lai. *Learning the Alexander Technique.* VHS. Venice, Calif.: VisionQuest Video, 1998.
The Alexander Technique was founded by Shakespearean actor Frederick Matthias Alexander, who was born in Tasmania in 1869. He discovered that unconscious movements during recitation caused him to lose his voice, and that realization lead him to study movement and develop his technique. Following the technique allows students to learn to release tension and reduce stress by avoiding unconscious misuse of the muscles of the body.

Gelb, Michael. *Putting Your Genius to Work.* Audio cassette tapes. Niles, Ill.: Nightingale-Conant Corp., 1996.
Components include "A New Renaissance," "The Secret to a Good Memory," "The Power of Creative Visualization," "Learning: The Art of Play," "How to Think Like Leonardo da Vinci," "Embracing Change with Synvergent Thinking," "Five Phases of Creative Problem Solving," "A Synvergent Approach to Fitness," "The Seven Principles of the Alexander Technique," "Becoming a Creativity Coach," and "An Interview with Michael Gelb."

A Holistic Approach to Arthritis Treatment: Building a Bridge between Conventional and Alternative Therapies. **VHS. Chicago: Arthritis Foundation, 1998.**
Discussion of the treatment of arthritis using both conventional and alternative methods. The alternative methods discussed include chiropractic, naprapathy, Chinese medicine, the Alexander Technique, and others.

Jordan, James Mark, and Heather Buchanan. ***Evoking Sound Body Mapping and Basic Conducting Techniques.*** **VHS. Chicago: GIA, 2002.**
Taking James Jordan's choral conducting book *Evoking Sound* to the next level, this video is a self-tutorial that demonstrates and enhances the basic conducting principles discussed in the book. This insightful presentation includes an overview of fundamental body mapping based upon the Alexander Technique as applied to choral conducting, as well as tutorials on breathing and basic conducting patterns.

Jourdy, Rafaele. ***The Head Leads and the Body Follows: An Introduction to the Alexander Technique.*** **VHS. Sydney, Australia: In Such a Way, 1996.**
Introduces the Alexander Technique, a movement education for the enhancement of personal performance. Not a "how to" video, since personal instruction is necessary to learn the technique.

Kingsley, Anthony P., Robin Ellis, and Robb Hart. ***From Stress to Freedom with the Alexander Technique.*** **VHS. London: Alexander Technique Center for Training and Development, 1990.**
Commentary and demonstration of the Alexander Technique to improve physical and mental functioning and reduce stress by preventing misuse of the body. The technique emphasizes directed relaxation and breathing exercises and concentrates on the interactions of head, neck, and back.

Kosminsky, Jane, and William Hurt. ***The Balance of Well-Being: The Alexander Technique.*** **VHS. New York: Balance of Well-Being, 1999.**

———. ***First Lesson: An Introduction to the Alexander Technique.*** **VHS. New York: Wellspring Media, 1999.**
William Hurt joins former dancer and certified Alexander teacher Jane Kosminsky in a pioneer videotape about the performer's secret weapon—the Alexander Technique. For over one hundred years the technique has helped performers to look better, breathe better, move better, and even bow better.

Kosminsky, Jane, et al. ***For Dancers: The Alexander Technique.*** **DVD. New York: Balance of Well-Being, 2005.**
The Alexander Technique in core movement, including alignment, plié, tendu, extension, bending, twisting, arms, and jumping. Includes a quick reference to the Alexander principles—a class: some unanswered questions, including breathing, how to sit on the floor, how to improve turnout, work on arabesque, a conversation with dancers, how Alexander Technique may be used in choreographic styles of Martha Graham, Bob Fosse, and William Forsythe, and so forth.

Learning the Alexander Technique. **VHS. Venice, Calif.: VisionQuest Home Media, 1998.**
Introduction to the technique, origin of this therapy, benefits of learning and practicing it; includes case examples and demonstrations.

Lim, Serene, Celia Tate, and Brian Beaton. *Movement.* **VHS. Falls Church, Va.: Landmark Media, 1996.**
Dr. Lim Serene shows how many conditions can be treated with movement therapies. Also in DVD (Falls Church, Va.: Landmark Media, 2004).

Master Class with Marjory Barlow. **VHS. Ojai, Calif.: Alexander Teaching Associates, 1988.**
During a session at the 1st International Alexander Congress, Marjory Barlow, niece of F. M. Alexander, demonstrates the Alexander Technique on a subject who is lying down.

McBride, Molly, William Hurt, Jane Kosminsky, and Deborah Caplan. *The Alexander Technique.* **DVD. New York: Wellspring Media, 2000.**
The Alexander Technique has been used for decades by dancers, actors, and singers to improve their performance, energy, and health. The first program shows the fundamentals, the second program illustrates special variations on the technique to effectively prevent or relieve back pain for good.

Moving Mindfully: A Self-help Guide to the Alexander Technique. **Compact disc. Florence, Mass.: AmSAT, 2003.**

Murdock, Ronald. *Voice and the Alexander Technique.* **Audio cassette tape. N.p.: Author, 1990–1994.**

Paige, Sheila, and Keith Mathis. *Piano Wellness Seminar: Innovations in Technique.* **DVD. Cherry Hill, N.J.: Piano Wellness, 2006.**
Ms. Paige has developed many new ideas based on her study of the Taubman technique, Alexander Technique, and other methods. This lecture includes her latest innovations, not found in any other setting.

Rubenfeld, Ilana, Arthur Bloch, and Jeffrey Mishlove. *Mind-Body Integration.* **VHS. Berkeley, Calif.: Thinking Allowed Productions, 1992.**
Explains the Rubenfeld Synergy Method, which incorporates elements of the Alexander Technique, Feldenkrais, gestalt psychotherapy, and Ericksonian hypnosis into one unique psychotherapeutic modality.

Sojkowski, Gary, and Marlies Yearby. *Talkin'.* **VHS. Becket, Mass.: Jacob's Pillow, 1991.**
Performed by Gary Sojkowski, Marlies Yearby, and students in the Jacob's Pillow new vision workshop. Videotaped in performance in the Studio Theater, Jacob's Pillow, Becket, Massachusetts, on August 4, 1991. The new vision work-

shop was aimed at developing a holistic view of dance through technique classes, improvisation, yoga, Alexander Technique, and other methods.

Stone, Robert B. *Mind/Body Communication*. Audio cassette tapes. Niles, Ill.: Nightingale-Conant Corp., 1993.
Components include "Mind/Body Communication: Why It Works," "Your Bones and the Alexander Technique," "A Fantastic Voyage," "Your Immune System and the Simonton Method," "The Incredible Power of Your Consciousness," "Reprogramming Yourself with Self-hypnotism," "Cyberphysiology and the Silva Method," "More Mind/Body Communication Techniques," "Cyberphysiology: A Resource for Creative Healing," "Healing Your Inner Self with Cyberphysiology," "Your On-going Good Health and Autogenic Training," and "Support Groups: Talking Health to One Another."

Tierney, Judy. *My Aching Back*. DVD. Sydney, Australia: ABC, 2005.
A general practitioner, acupuncturist, and Alexander Technique specialist discusses complementary treatment for chronic back pain. Case studies.

8

Directory of
Alexander Technique Associations

This chapter provides a directory of Alexander Technique teacher training schools and associations in the English-speaking world, including the United States, Canada, Australia, and Great Britain. Teacher training schools provide instruction for the certification of professionals who want to teach Alexander Technique lessons to individuals. Most Alexander Technique professional associations emphasize the importance of taking lessons with a certified teacher. This training requires more than 1,600 hours of classes over at least a three-year period. For each entry, a director of the school has been listed unless that school's website lists only faculty members and does not designate a director. Where the school has a small faculty, these teachers have been listed, but for schools with a large faculty, no contact name has been given. For some entries, e-mail address was not available on the school's website. Refer to the Web page for electronic communication in these instances. Some schools do not have a permanent physical address, offering classes in local facilities that have other purposes as well, such as churches and colleges. For these schools, only phone, e-mail, and website have been provided.

UNITED STATES

The Alexander Alliance
Director: Bruce Fertman
605 West Phil Ellena Street
Philadelphia, PA 19119
Phone: 215-844-0670 or 215-386-9705
E-mail: AlliancePhilly@aol.com
www.alexanderalliance.com/

Alexander Alliance schools also in Coyote, N.Mex.; Kyoto, Japan; Tokyo, Japan; Toronto, Canada; and several locations in Germany (contact available on main website)

The Alexander Educational Center
Directors: Giora Pinkas and John Baron
2727 College Avenue
Berkeley, CA 94705
Phone: 925-933-0602
E-mail: info@alexandertechnique.org
www.alexandertechnique.org/

The Alexander Technique Center at Cambridge
Director: Tommy Thompson
1692 Massachusetts Avenue, 3rd Floor
Cambridge, MA 02138
Phone: 617-497-2242
E-mail: info@ATCambridge.com
www.easeofbeing.com/training.htm

The Alexander Technique Connexion New England
94 Lessey Street
Amherst, MA 01002
Phone: 413-253-2595
E-mail: info@atcne.com
www.atcne.com/

The Alexander Technique Moving Arts Centre
Director: Sumi Komo
1406-F Oxford Avenue
Austin, TX 78704
Phone: 512-448-4009
www.alexandermovingarts.com/

Alexander Technique New York
Faculty: John Nicholls and Nanette Walsh
19 West 34th Street #1013
(between 5th and 6th Avenues)
New York, NY 10001
Phone: 212-706-2507
E-mail: info@atnyc.us
www.atnyc.us/index_files/Page601.htm

Alexander Technique Training Center
Director: Ruth Kilroy
701 Beacon Street
Newton Center, MA 02459
Phone: 617-641-0048
E-mail: ruthattc@yahoo.com
www.attcboston.com/

Alexander Technique Urbana
608 E. Burkwood Ct.
Urbana, IL 61801
Directors: Rose Bronec and Rick Carbaugh
Phone: 217-344-5274
E-mail: rbronec@synidetics.com
www.synidetics.com/

Alexander Training Institute of Los Angeles
1526 14th Street #110
Santa Monica, CA 90025
Phone: 310-395-9170
E-mail: ATInstituteLA@aol.com
www.atinstitutela.com/

American Center for the Alexander Technique
Director: Joan Frost
39 West 14th Street, Room 507
(between 5th and 6th Avenues)
New York, NY 10011
Phone: 212-633-2229
www.acatnyc.org/teacher_certification_program.html

The Bay Area Center for the Alexander Technique
Director: Jerry Sontag
2560 9th Street, Studio 123A
Berkeley, CA 94710-2581
Phone: 510-486-1317
E-mail: Alexander@mtpress.com
www.mtpress.com/training.htm

North Carolina Alexander Technique Program
Director: Robin Gilmore
1204 Oak Hill Place #2C
Annapolis, MD 21403
Phone: 410-268-2841
E-mail: rglimmer@mindspring.com
www.alexandertechnique.com/robingilmore/

The Performance School
Faculty: Catherine Kettrick, David M. Mills, and Stacy Gehman
6836 21st Avenue NE
Seattle, WA 98115
Phone: 206-522-3584
www.performanceschool.org/

The Philadelphia School for the Alexander Technique
Director: Martha Fertman
Phone: 215-219-8594
http://phillyATtraining.googlepages.com

CANADA

Toronto School of the Alexander Technique
Faculty: Elaine Kopman and Howard Bockner
620 Wilson Avenue, Suite 210
Toronto, ON M3K 1Z3
Phone: 416-631-8127
E-mail: info@alexandertechnique.ca
www.alexandertechnique.ca/

The Vancouver School for the Alexander Technique
Codirector: Gabriella Minnes Brandes
4125 Heather Street
Vancouver, BC V5Z 4H1
Phone: 604-737-2818
E-mail: gaby@interchange.ubc.ca
http://members.shaw.ca/AlexanderTechniqueTraining/

UNITED KINGDOM

The Alexander Technique College
Director: Carolyn Nicholls
Unit 3, Hove Business Centre, Fonthill Road
Brighton, East Sussex BN3 6HA
Phone: 01273 562595
E-mail: carolyn.nicholls@alexander-technique-college.com
www.alexander-technique-college.com/

The Alexander Technique Teacher Training School
Head of Training: Anthony Kingsley
1st floor, Danceworks
16 Balderton Street
London W1K 6TN
Phone: 02076 291808
E-mail: enquiries@alexanderteacher.co.uk
www.alexanderteacher.co.uk/

The Bristol Alexander Technique Training School Association
Director: Caroline Chalk
Long Ashton Guides HQ
Weston Road
Long Ashton
Bristol BS41 9BJ
Phone: 01761 439904
E-mail: cchalk@onetel.net
www.battsa.co.uk/

Constructive Teaching Centre
Directors: Dilys Carrington and Ruth Murray
18 Lansdowne Road
Holland Park
London W11 3LL
Phone: 02077 277222
E-mail: info@alexandertek.com
www.alexandertek.com/

Essex Alexander School
Director: Ken Thompson
65 Norfolk Road
Seven Kings
Ilford, Essex 1G3 8LJ
Phone: 02082 201630
E-mail: ken_thompson@lineone.net
www.essexalexanderschool.co.uk/

Interactive Teaching Method Association
Director: Tracy Gil
PO Box 181
Bristol BS99 7BH
Phone: 08451 298395
www.alexandertechnique-itm.org/

The Manchester Alexander Technique Training School
Director: Malcolm Williamson
c/o Royal Northern College of Music
124 Oxford Road
Manchester M13 9RD
Phone: 01612 241112
E-mail: williamm@rncm.ac.uk
www.alextechteaching.org.uk/

AUSTRALIA

The Alexander Technique Institute
Director: Diana Devitt-Dawson
Suite 4, 188 Pacific Highway
North Sydney, NSW 2060
Phone: 61 2 9955 0110
E-mail: diana@alexandertechniqueinstitute.com.au
www.alexandertechniqueinstitute.com.au/

The School for F. M. Alexander Studies
Director: David Moore
330 St. Georges Road (corner of Holden Street)
North Fitzroy, Victoria 3068
Phone: 61 3 9486 5900
E-mail: info@alexanderschool.edu.au
www.alexanderschool.edu.au/

A Brief Glossary of Significant Terms

body mapping. This is a term that was not in use by F. M. Alexander, but it has come into considerable usage since it was coined by Alexander teachers Barbara and William Conable. Body mapping refers to a person's perceived view of their own body, how it is shaped, its size, how the body moves, and how it functions. People can have a good or bad perception of their body map. When it is good, the person moves with poise and balance.

conscious control. This is the way individuals think about their habitual use of their body once they become aware of their habits of misuse, inhibit those habits, and then process mental directions to relearn movement of use. Conscious control is needed to overcome habits of misuse and is achieved when individuals are able to knowingly change their habits of misuse regularly.

direction/directions. There are two uses of these terms in the Alexander Technique, but they are directly linked to each other. First, directions are the mental instructions one uses to undo habits of misuse and do learned actions that reduce unwanted tensions. These mental directions are needed to achieve conscious control over the automatic habits that cause tension. Second, this term is used to indicate the direction to release and lengthen muscles.

doing. In Alexander Technique circles, "doing" is considered a negative action. This refers to the tendency to make our muscles move physically rather than thinking the directions that will change the way the muscles are used. This is usually so with novice learners and relates to the process of "end-gaining."

end-gaining. In Alexander Technique circles, "end-gaining" is considered a negative action. End-gaining is the tendency, some say universal tendency, to focus our thoughts and actions on the end result of what we want to achieve. Alexander found that, by focusing on the result, it was very difficult to go through the process of learning conscious control.

faulty sensory awareness. When the body moves, the individual senses how the body is being used and what is happening with the movement. Habits of misuse send faulty signals about how the body is actually being used. The individual perceives that it is good and comfortable, for example. Alexander called this his "debauched kinesthesia."

going-up. This is a specialized term within the Alexander Technique context. It refers to how the body is organized in relation to the crown of the head. It is considered a thought process rather than a physical activity.

inhibition. This is the concept that the individual, after becoming aware of a habit of misuse, uses a thought process to stop, or inhibit, a habitual reaction to a stimulus that causes a specific movement. This thought process of stopping the habitual reaction allows the individual to choose to undo or substitute a learned response to that reaction, often done in a split second of time.

kinesthetic sense. All individuals will respond to a stimulus that corresponds to movement in the body. For example, it may be a visual image, such as a green light when driving that makes you move your foot on the gas peddle. It may also be verbal, such as when you are startled by a sharp, unexpected sound that makes you jump out of your seat. Kinesthetic sense is what gives us information about our body and its movement, and whether or not our different body parts move easily or with difficulty.

lengthening. Generally, this refers to when a specific muscle is increased in length. In the Alexander Technique, this refers to utilizing the full length of the spine without straining or forcing it to lengthen.

means-whereby. This term was used by Alexander to describe how we use our body when doing any activity. As students work to obtain conscious control, they are instructed to consider the "means-whereby" of their movement. When the individual can realize this "means-whereby," they can employ mental directions to react in new ways of movement.

misuse. This term has a specific context within the Alexander Technique. Misuse is an inappropriate use of the body, often habitually, that causes some harm or potentially causes some harm, loss of balance and poise, muscle tone, coordination, and other concerns.

nondoing. This term is unique to the Alexander Technique, and in Alexander Technique circles, this is a desirable process. Nondoing refers to thinking about a goal rather than making it happen by physically trying to realize that goal. Nondoing needs to be achieved to overcome end-gaining.

primary control. As explained above, this term is a specific concept unique to the Alexander Technique. Alexander used this term to label the relationship of the head to the neck, and the position of the head and neck to the rest of the torso or body. It is more than just the position of these body features. Primary control is a balanced relationship between the head, neck, and torso. Primary control is what will be achieved when the four mental directions, described above, are working well.

proprioception. The American Heritage® Science Dictionary, from Dictionary.com website, at http://dictionary.reference.com/browse/proprioception (accessed November 6, 2007), defines this term as follows: "The unconscious perception of movement and spatial orientation arising from stimuli within the body itself. In humans, these stimuli are detected by nerves within the body itself, as well as by the semicircular canals of the inner ear."

think-up. This is a specialized term within the Alexander Technique context. It is the same as and interchangeable with the term "going-up." It refers to how the body is organized in relation to the crown of the head. It is considered a thought process rather than a physical activity.

use. This term, as used by the Alexander Technique, refers to how we habitually use our body for movement. The manner in which we use ourselves impacts how the whole body behaves or functions.

Author Index

Subject Index

About the Authors

John B. Harer is assistant professor of library science at East Carolina University, Greenville, N.C. He earned his PhD in Educational Administration from Texas A&M University and his master's in library science from Clarion University of Pennsylvania. He is the author of several books on intellectual freedom, including the resource book *Intellectual Freedom: A Reference Handbook* (1992), and numerous articles on intellectual freedom, storytelling, and library services.

Sharon Munden is associate professor of vocal studies and chair of the Department of Vocal Studies at East Carolina University, Greenville, N.C. A mezzo-soprano, she has performed on the opera stage at numerous international and national performances including at the LaScala, Milan, Italy; Spoleto Festival, Italy; Chamber Opera Theatre of New York; Chautauqua Opera; Fort Worth Opera; Glimmerglass Opera; Greater Miami Opera; Minnesota Opera; and Sarasota Opera. She is currently in teacher training for the Alexander Technique under the tutelage of Bruce Fertman and Martha Hansen Fertman.

ML

$\frac{5}{09}$